SELF-INJURIOUS BEHAVIOR

A Somatosensory
Treatment Approach

Haru Hirama, Ed.D., O.T.R./L.

ISBN 0-935273-01-8

Published by CHESS Publications, Inc., (301) 243-5943
Business Office: 232 East University Parkway, Baltimore, MD 21218
Editorial Office: 6007 Beech Avenue, Bethesda, MD 20817

Printed in the United States of America

DEDICATION

This is dedicated to the memory of my mother, Kiyoshi Ogasawara Hirama, and father, Soju Hirama. Images of my childhood kept entering my mind as I read about self-injurious behavior, and as I observed patients engaged in the behavior. Somehow my mother knew the importance of somatosensory stimulation. It seemed she concentrated on tactile stimulation, and my father provided activities for vestibular, proprioceptive, and kinesthetic stimulation. My mother prepared the furo for the family to soak to their chin in hot water each night. Lotion was not to be lightly smeared on the skin, but needed to be massaged with deep, long strokes along muscle fibers. Using deep massage, she rubbed away my annual green apple stomachaches during my single-digit years. She rubbed away pain in my legs. When I could not sleep, she lightly scratched my back until I fell asleep.

iii

ACKNOWLEDGEMENTS

I thank the late Margaret Grandovic, former Coordinator of the Special Education Program at Lehigh University's College of Education, for encouraging me to continue my study of self-injurious behavior; Elvin G. Warfel, Coordinator of the Teacher Education Program at Lehigh University's College of Education for supervising my research and dissertation and for his continued kindness and interest in my professional pursuits; Linda Kent, former Director of Occupational Therapy at Hunterdon Developmental Center, and her staff, who made possible the research related in Chapter 3; Steven C. Hayes, Department of Psychology, University of Nevada-Reno, who helped write Chapter 3; and the parents of patients who permitted me to work with their children.

PREFACE

I have hesitated writing this book because I know that self-injurious behavior needs further careful research. However, each time I see another self-injurious individual and the dilemma and frustration imposed upon teachers and therapists who must do something for the welfare of that individual, I want to let them know what has worked for me. Much of what I present as treatment is based on empirical data. My readings lead me to believe that future research will show some scientific basis for what I propose. I also believe that treatment is most effective when science and art are combined.

I am proposing a very practical treatment in which stimulation is given to counteract the somatosensory deprivation experienced by the self-injurious individual. As the self-injurious behavior decreases, the individual is manually guided to assist in his or her self-care. Eating, washing hands and face, brushing teeth, brushing hair, and other self-care tasks will gradually improve and self-injury will decrease and eventually be inhibited. It is because I have been in the same situation as those people involved in the care and education of these individuals that I share the information that follows.

CONTENTS

Chapter I

DESCRIPTION AND ETIOLOGY

Darlene is a nonverbal, nonambulatory, blind, institutionalized 10-year-old who looks as though she was beaten. Her eyes are swollen shut and the surrounding skin is discolored with bruises.

Mary is a nonverbal, nonambulatory, institutionalized 12-year-old. Her arms and legs are covered with scratches, some bleeding, some coated with scabs. Her scalp has numerous open scratches and bald spots.

Brian is a nonverbal, nonambulatory, institutionalized nine-year-old. His large, distended abdomen on a thin body gives an appearance similar to that of malnourished children. Brian's condition is caused by swallowing air (aerophagia).

Edna is a nonverbal institutionalized, nonambulatory 19-year-old. She is restrained in a heavy canvas jacket with wooden slats in the sleeves to keep her elbows extended. Cotton mittens are tied around her wrists. If left unrestrained, she bangs her head, hits her arms, legs, and face, and scratches inside her mouth until she bleeds.

In some institutions, some individuals have been restrained for most of the day with ankles and wrists tied to the four corners of a crib in "spread-eagle" fashion to prevent self-injury.

These are a few examples of individuals with self-inflicted injury treated by the author. The cause of this behavior is unclear. The seriousness of self-injury is evident from reports of at least one death from severe head banging that precipitated an intracranial hemorrhage, detached retinas, enucleation, laceration, and infection of open wounds (Mikkelsen, 1986).

Preferred Term

Various terms are used to label the behavior due to the lack of agreement on the etiology of self-inflicted injury. Self-mutilative behavior (Crabtree, 1967; Lester, 1972; Mizuno and Yugari, 1975); self-abusive behavior (Mantione, 1977); auto-erotic and tantrum head banging (Silberstein, Blackman and Mandell, 1966); and self-injurious behavior (Tate and Baroff, 1966) have been used synonymously.

In this text, self-injurious behavior (SIB) will be used throughout, even though authors whose works are cited may have used one of the above terms to refer to the behavior. Tate and Baroff (1966) state that SIB is a descriptive phrase denoting behavior which results in physical injury. It does not imply willful intention to injure oneself nor suggest other interpretations of the behavior. SIB seems to be the current preferred term.

Incidence

Incidences of SIB have been reported in normal children. The highest reported incidence of 11 to 17 percent occurred during the ages of 19 to 32 months (DeLissovoy, 1963). Normal children were found to be free of SIB by five years of age. Five percent more boys than girls were involved in SIB in the normal population (Lourie, 1949).

SIB has been most frequently seen in individuals classified as mentally retarded or mentally ill. A 3.4 percent incidence was reported among the mentally ill population, and a 15 percent incidence was reported among the mentally retarded population (Williams, 1974). The ratio of SIB was one male to three females in children diagnosed as schizophrenic. The SIB persisted in the mentally ill and mentally retarded population beyond the five years of age at which time SIB disappeared in normal children (Green, 1967).

Carr (1977) reported that five hypotheses were most frequently cited as motivational variables of SIB: the positive reinforcement hypothesis, the negative reinforcement hypothesis, the self-stimulation hypothesis, the organic hypothesis, and the psychodynamic hypothesis.

The positive reinforcement hypothesis states that SIB is a learned operant, maintained by positive social reinforcement (Lovaas, Freitag, Gold and Kassorla, 1965). This hypothesis suggests that after an individual has displayed SIB, the response to the behavior by those individuals in the environment has a rewarding and reinforcing effect on the behavior. It is further suggested that when the social consequences that presumably maintain the behavior are withdrawn, the frequency of SIB will decrease.

The negative reinforcement hypothesis states that SIB is maintained by the termination or avoidance of an aversive stimulus following the occurrence of a self-injurious act (Carr, Newsom, and Binkoff, 1976). The literature supporting this hypothesis demonstrates the role of escape factors as the motivation maintaining SIB.

The self-stimulation hypothesis presumes that certain levels of somatosensory stimulation, primarily in the tactile, vestibular and kinesthetic modalities, are necessary for the human organism. When somatosensory stimulation is inadequate, the organism may engage in stereotyped behavior, including SIB, as a means of providing its own sensory stimulation (Baumeister and Forehand, 1973; Cain, 1961; Cleland and Clark, 1966; Green, 1967; Kukla, Fry and Goldstein, 1960; Lourie, 1949; Rutter, 1966, p. 80; Silberstein, Blackman and Mandell, 1966). Studies with primates (Harlow and Harlow, 1962) have shown that many of the partially isolated monkeys engaged in a variety of repetitive, stereotyped acts, such as rocking, cage circling, staring into space and SIB in the form of self-biting. Monkeys reared with their mothers rarely exhibited these behaviors. One interpretation is that cage-reared isolates, being deprived of tactile and kinesthetic stimulation, generate their own stimulation, through stereotyped, repetitive behavior as well as through SIB.

The organic hypothesis states that SIB is a product of aberrant physiological processes. Reported studies postulating an organic cause involve the syndromes of Lesch-Nyhan, XXXXY Chromosomal, and deLange, and the medical problem of otitis media (Lesch and Nyhan, 1964).

The psychodynamic hypothesis states that SIB is an attempt to establish ego boundaries or to reduce guilt (Carr, 1977). SIB is hypothesized as being an attempt to establish "body reality" (Greenacre in Carr, 1977); to trace "ego boundaries" (Hartman, Kres and Loewenstein, in Carr, 1977); or "body boundaries" (Bychowski, in Carr, 1977). Green (1967) reviewed some psychodynamic hypotheses in SIB. Spitz and Wolfe (in Green, 1967) explained head banging and other SIB in infants as the infant's aggressive and libidinal drives being turned inward when no external object was available. Anna Freud distinguished between self-injury in children, believed to be due to a maturational defect, and later aggression turned toward the self, believed to be a defense mechanism used by the ego under the pressure of conflict (Green, 1967). Lester (1972) believes anger plays a role in SIB. Anger which cannot be expressed outwardly is believed to be turned inward.

The etiology of SIB is still undetermined. It is likely that a variety of factors are responsible for SIB.

Chapter II

LITERATURE REVIEW
OF TREATMENT

The shocking and repugnant nature of self-injurious behavior (SIB) often forces caretakers to stop the behavior by any available method. A review of reported treatment methods follows.

Restraints

Physical restraints have commonly been used to prevent SIB (Bachman, 1972; Baumeister and Baumeister, 1978; Birnbauer, 1968; Picker, Poling and Parker, 1979; Stainback, Stainback and Dedrick, 1979; Tate and Baroff, 1966; Weiher and Harman, 1975). In most studies reported, the subject had been routinely placed in restraints prior to the study.

Weiher and Harman (1975) stated that their subject had routinely been placed in a chair at the beginning of each day and strapped at the waist and chest. The chair had padded panels extending on each side of the subject's head to prevent striking his head on the nearby surfaces. The subject was taken out of the chair only during baths, diaper changes, and occasional naps in bed. The subject was maintained in this pattern of restraint for two and one-half years prior to the study.

Luiselli (1986) successfully modified SIB in a 16½-year-old, deaf, blind, developmentally disabled male by the contingent use of a padded helmet and mittens. When SIB occurred, the staff member stopped the behavior, applied the protective equipment, and had the subject sit in the nearest chair. The equipment remained in place until the SIB was absent for 30 seconds while the subject remained seated in the chair. When the 30-second criterion was reached, the subject was guided out of the chair, the equipment was removed, and he resumed the scheduled activity. This procedure was coupled with a reinforcement program in which the staff member interacted with the subject by tactually signing "good boy—no hitting (banging)" and gave him desired edible items for each 15 minutes of no SIB.

From the 23rd day of treatment, the time interval for reinforcement was gradually increased and was discontinued on day 58. Staff members used physical touch and other means of praise for behaviors other than SIB. Initial baseline responses recorded were 7.9 each hour, compared to 1.4 per hour at the end of the treatment program and 0.25 responses per hour at the 6-month follow-up assessment.

Some subjects were reported to have been fully restrained (Myers and Deibert, 1971) or fully restrained in bed (Merbaum, 1973; Romanczyk and Goren, 1975; Tate and Baroff, 1966) for as long as four years. Tanner and Zeiler (1975) reported that prior to their study the subject wore a padded helmet all day and occasionally had both arms tied to the chair. Saposnek and Watson (1974) described their subject as having both arms restrained while awake and asleep.

One subject was physically restrained at all times with splints and restraint jacket and with legs fastened to the chair legs (Mutter, Pick, Whitlow and Fraser, 1975). Tate (1972) reported on a subject who had been restrained in bed for seven and one-half years. The subject's legs were padded with four-inch thick polyurethane foam. A two-inch thick polyurethane foam collar was placed around the neck, and wrist cuffs were applied and fastened to the bed. The fingers were taped and cotton mitts were securely taped on at the wrist. The subject had bitten her lips, so all of her teeth had been removed.

Lane and Dormath (1970) stated that restraining by tying the individual to a chair was extremely aversive and was not a rapid form of treatment to reduce SIB. Jacobs, Lynch, Cornick, and Slifer (1986) found mechanical restraints or restraining in a chair increased aggression in a 14-year-old aggressive and self-injurious male with Reye's syndrome. A contingent restraint procedure was used in which one or more staff members placed the patient supine and manually restrained him by the arms, trunk, and legs. If the patient remained calm for one minute, he was allowed to resume previous activities. SIB disappeared, as this treatment reduced the aggressive behavior.

The patient's hands held on his knees by the therapist while he was seated in a chair worked successfully with a 14-year-old profoundly retarded, noninstitutionalized male, who displayed SIB of slapping and punching his head and biting his fingers and hands. The SIB was often accompanied by screaming, jumping, running, and clinging to the nearest person. The behavior resulted in suspension from the special school. Treatment was given in three settings: (1) toilet cubicle with two chairs, toys, and cleaning equipment; (2) a small teaching room with two chairs, two tables, toys, and office equipment; and (3) a large classroom with other children and classroom equipment. The treatment sessions were three times a day for a total of two and one-half hours per day over five school days. Number of days for setting 1 was 27; for setting 2, 18 days; and for setting 3, 18 days. Treatment consisted of a verbal prompt to sit on a chair and calm down. If he did not, he was manually guided to sit, and his hands were held on his knees by the therapist while he was told to keep his hands away from his head. When his hands relaxed, the therapist released his hands. The treatment was repeated if SIB resumed. If there was no SIB, he was given eight ounces of orange juice and verbal praise (Tierney, 1986).

Williams (1974) stated that he had success with an autistic woman who ceased to damage her face after wearing a fencing mask continuously for two weeks. This enabled the staff to engage her in activities so the SIB did not recur. Azrin, Gottlieb, Hughart, Wesolowski, and Rahn (1975) found that some of the subjects in their study seemed to prefer being restrained and would self-injure in an effort to be put in physical restraints. Buchar and Lovaas (1968), and Lovaas and Simmons (1969), found some individuals became accustomed to being in restraints, and removal of the restraints caused a dramatic increase in SIB.

Schroeder, Peterson, Solomon, and Artley (1977) studied three conditions using restraints to reduce head banging in two severely mentally retarded adolescent males. Restraints for SIB and verbal reinforcement for relaxation were effective in reducing head banging. Restraints for SIB and verbal reinforcement and EMG biofeedback were more effective than without EMG biofeedback. Verbal and edible reinforcements for relaxation were more effective than verbal reinforcement alone. Restraints have been the most widely used form of treatment to prevent SIB, and it may be necessary to gradually eliminate their use. Corbett (1975) reported that Williams, in a paper presented at the Ninth International Study Group on Child Neurology and Cerebral Palsy, at Oxford, gave an account of a splint made from copies of *The Times*, which was gradually removed page by page over a period of time without recurrence of head banging in the subject. Dorsey, Iwata, Reid, and Davis (1982) showed reduction in head hitting, eye gouging, and hand biting in three teenage retarded clients with use of contingent application of

padded gloves and football helmet. They state that such protective equipment seems justified when compared to aversive procedures in use. A variety of physical restraints used to prevent SIB have been described; however, adequate numbers of well-designed studies have not been conducted to establish the efficacy of physical restraints in extinguishing SIB.

Psychodynamic Treatment

Treatment based on the hypothesis that psychodynamic factors are the underlying motive for SIB has been infrequently reported. Picker, Poling and Parker (1979) stated that psychoanalytical explanations have not been directly testable nor have they fostered viable treatments.

Green (1967) commented that his findings showing the wide prevalence of SIB in the group of schizophrenic children compared to the absence of SIB in normal children of the same age was one aspect of the ego impairment found in childhood schizophrenia. The disordered body image, the inability to differentiate self from nonself, and the faulty perceptions and integration of painful stimuli were believed to form the matrix in which SIB develops. Lovaas, Freitag, Gold, and Kassorla (1965) included in their study an attempt to alleviate guilt in a self-injurious child by making statements such as, "I don't think you're bad," each time the child hit herself. The statements increased the SIB, thus, were considered reinforcing rather than guilt-alleviating.

Crabtree (1967) reported having successfully eliminated SIB in a 16-year-old female through psychotherapy. The patient began scratching herself with a pin when a male teacher failed to give her the attention she desired. The behavior attracted his attention, but the teacher expressed anger at the SIB. Psychotherapy revealed that the patient had a strong desire to be close to others. The patient revealed fantasies of being beaten and smashed. A strong sense of badness and fearfulness was also expressed by the patient. The scratching was reported to have been extinguished through continued psychotherapy and by teaching the patient cognitive control over her SIB.

Carr (1977) pointed out the difficulty in operationalizing constructs such as "ego impairment," "body reality," "ego boundaries," and "guilt" upon which the psychodynamic hypotheses are based. The lack of operational constructs prevents the hypothesis from being adequately tested.

Chemotherapy

SIB, which has been believed to be based in aberrant physiological processes, has been treated by specific chemicals, combinations of chemicals, medical, and surgical procedures. Most frequently reported physiological conditions which included SIB in the symptoms were the Lesch-Nyhan syndrome, the deLange syndrome, and otitis media.

The Lesch-Nyhan syndrome has been classified as an X-linked form of cerebral palsy found in males. A flaw in purine metabolism results in a deficiency of the enzyme hypoxanthine-quanine phosphoribosyltransferase. Reported characteristics displayed by individuals with this syndrome include muscle spasticity, choreoathetosis, mental retardation, hyperuricemia, and SIB. The SIB most often seen has been in the form of compulsive, repetitive biting of the tongue, lips, and fingers (Lesch and Nyhan, 1964). Seegmiller, Rosenbloom, and Kelley (1967) proposed that the SIB is directly produced by the resulting biochemical imbalance. Hoefnagel (1965) proposed that the irritation resulting from an elevated uric acid level in the saliva might explain why the SIB was directed to the tongue and lips.

Mizuno and Yugari (1974) reported success in eliminating SIB with L-5-hydroxytryptophan. In 1976, Nyhan reported inability to control SIB with L-5-hydroxytryptophan. These conflicting reports added to the question of whether SIB in the Lesch-Nyhan syndrome was actually due to the elevated uric acid levels. Duker (1975) successfully treated self-biting in a 15-year-old profoundly mentally retarded female diagnosed with Lesch-Nyhan syndrome using time out from social reinforcement. Duker's successful treatment raised questions as to the organic basis of SIB in Lesch-Nyhan syndrome.

Two studies (Sandman et al., 1983; Davidson et al., 1983) reported success in reducing SIB in three mentally retarded males by using naloxone. Naloxone is an opiate antagonist used by some researchers who reason that individuals with severe SIB do not experience pain as most people do. Another study (Beckwith et al., 1986) using naloxone to reduce SIB in two developmentally delayed females was not successful. Both females had seizures; one was deaf and blind, the second was diagnosed with phenylketonuria.

Baumeister and Rollings (1976) proposed that SIB in the deLange syndrome individual may be a behavioral manifestation of the organic disease. They suggested that SIB may be seizure-like episodes which were triggered by either structural or chemical defects in the brain.

Mikkelsen (1986) successfully reduced SIB in five females ranging in age from 19 to 34 and one 40-year-old male with a low-dose haloperidol treatment program. After treatment was started the individuals were described as appearing more healthy, more alert, and more focused, with longer attention spans. The length of follow-up was six months for two patients, more than one year for three patients, and over five years for one.

Peterson and Peterson (1968) conducted a three-part experimental study on an eight-year-old mentally retarded boy with SIB. Their subject was receiving thioridazine hydrochloride and chlorpromazine prior to and during most of the study. There seemed to be no relationship between the presence or absence of the medication and the rate of SIB. Results of the reversal period in their study showed the medications were not responsible for the changes in SIB. Lovaas and Simon (1969) stated their subject had been on a combination of tranquilizers prior to their study with no visible effects. Reported results of the effect of chemicals and medical or surgical procedures on SIB have not clarified the effectiveness of those procedures.

Singh and Pullman (1979) treated a severely retarded 13-year-old male diagnosed as deLange syndrome. The subject's SIB included head and face slapping of at least three years' duration. Positive reinforcement was given initially for one-minute periods of no SIB. Gradually reinforcement was given for 30-minute periods of no SIB. Since SIB was not extinguished, a reversal period reestablished baseline and punishment was added to the first procedure. SIB was decreased 99.92 percent. Shear, Nyhan, Kirman, and Stern (1971) reported that the aversive stimulation was useful in controlling SIB in one deLange syndrome child whom they studied.

Primrose (1979) reported on a study which was based on the premise that SIB patients have a defect in the cortex or basal ganglia and might be deficient in a chemical required to inhibit certain impulses arising from these areas. Baclofen, a gamma-amino butyric acid (GABA) analogue that crosses the blood-brain barrier, was administered to 20 subjects with IQs less than 50 and with a variety of other disorders. Two subjects had phenylketonuria, a metabolic disorder in which the enzyme phenylalanine hydroxylase is absent and prevents the oxidation of phenylalanine to tyrosine. Sixteen of the subjects were epileptic, five subjects were blind, two subjects were deaf, and 19 subjects had no speech. During treatment, seizures increased in one subject but SIB decreased. Seizures were precipitated in another subject, so treatment was stopped. Anorexia, vomiting, loss of sphincter control, and drowsiness were other side effects from the GABA. General ratings of better, same, or worse behavior were obtained. Fourteen subjects were reported to have improved. A double blind test, in which a placebo and baclofen were administered for eight weeks each, resulted in no significant difference in 22 subjects; and in nine subjects improvement was seen after removal of the drug. The researcher concluded a form of behavior modification had taken place. Difficulty in analyzing the data was indicated.

De Lissovoy (1963) found a higher incidence of otitis media, a middle ear infection, in head bangers, and concluded head banging was a form of pain relief. The reports did not include conclusions on the effect of treatment of otitis media on SIB in these head bangers.

Neurosurgery

Reports of neurosurgical procedures to reduce SIB have not been encouraging. Reports often provided little detail of the patients involved. Corbett (1975) reviewed the results of surgical treatment by three separate research groups. One group reported one of five patients showed improvement and two of the five developed seizures postoperatively. A second group concluded surgical intervention was particularly disappointing in the severely retarded. The third group of surgeons found long-term results to be disappointing. Without clear evidence of the centers and connections in the brain involved in SIB, neurosurgical intervention cannot at present be considered a feasible treatment.

Sensory Stimulation

The self-stimulation hypothesis has been cited by many authors mentioned in this chapter. However, the literature on treatment of SIB using sensory stimulation procedures is sparse (Bailey and Meyerson, 1970; Bright, Bittick, and Kleeman, 1981; Lemke, 1974; and Wells and Smith, 1983). Carr (1977) reported some studies which were relevant to the hypothesis but stated the studies were inconclusive due to flaws in research methodology. In the 1965 studies by Hollis, head banging was included with behaviors such as complex hand movements and rocking, which did not result in self-injury. Carr stated that in Myerson, Kerr, and Michael's study, the treatment using vibration lasted for only two sessions and should be considered inconclusive.

A review of treatments by Picker et al. (1979) did not mention any studies in which sensory stimulation was used.

Behavior Modification

Most of the published research on treatment of SIB has been based on the hypothesis that SIB is a learned behavior and is contingent on external reinforcement (Carr, 1977; Picker et al., 1979; Smolev, 1971). A variety of techniques based on learning theory have been used by researchers to successfully reduce SIB. These techniques have been classified as extinction, positive reinforcement, negative reinforcement, punishment, and differential reinforcement of other or alternative behaviors.

Extinction

Extinction has been defined as a procedure which decreased the probability of a behaviors occurring by withholding the response-produced consequences. The undesirable behavior is extinguished by withdrawing the reinforcement which was maintaining it. Since SIB was believed to be maintained by social reinforcement, the technique used in extinction was to ignore the SIB.

Lovaas and Simmons (1969) used extinction procedures with an 11-year-old severely retarded boy. Restraints were removed, and the subject was isolated in a room so he could respond freely. SIB was reduced over 50 sessions from over 9,000 self-injurious responses (SIRs) per session to 30 SIRs per session. The researchers also studied a seven-year-old severely retarded boy in an extinction situation. The subject was left in his crib without restraints and allowed to bang his head against the crib and beat his head with his fist. By the tenth session extinction occurred, but the subject had hit himself approximately 9,000 times during those ten sessions.

In both cases, extinction was specific to the situation. Although SIB fell to zero in the experimental room, SIB remained unaffected in other situations, such as being held on the nurse's lap. A phenomenon known as "extinction burst," reported by Skinner (1938, p. 74, in Lovaas and Simmons, 1969) was also reported by the researchers. When the extinction procedure was initially begun, there was an acceleration in the number of self-injurious responses. The researchers concluded that extinction procedures would be effective if given sufficient time.

The procedure was not advised for children whose SIB posed a risk of severe or fatal damage. Use of the procedure would be difficult to defend ethically or legally when the enforced isolation and danger to the subject was considered (Picker et al., 1979; Smolev, 1971).

Positive Reinforcement

Treatment based on positive reinforcement hypothesizes that SIB was maintained by social reinforcement which was given the individual upon emission of the SIB. If SIB has not been reinforced by attention and periods of non-SIB were reinforced, the SIB should disappear.

Lovaas et al. (1965) were able to control the frequency of SIB in a nine-year-old girl diagnosed as schizophrenic with autistic and symbiotic features. The subject's SIB began at age three years. The behavior was primarily head banging and arm banging against furniture and walls and pinching and slapping herself. The subject was taught to clap and rock in time to music by giving social approval such as smiles and comments of "That's a good girl." The researchers showed that they could alternately increase appropriate music behavior and decrease SIB by giving approval for music behavior, and increase SIB and decrease appropriate music behavior by giving attention to SIB and ignoring appropriate music behavior. The same subject was taught bar-pressing following procedures similar to those in the first study. This study confirmed the findings of the first study. In a third study with the same subject, the comment, "I don't think you are bad," was said in a reassuring manner following the subject's SIB. This comment served as a reinforcer and increased the subject's SIB.

Repp and Deitz (1974) reinforced with candy periods of no SIB and successfully reduced SIB and aggressive behavior in four institutionalized individuals. Previous attempts to control the SIB by saying, "No!" pushing the subject's hand away, or ignoring the behavior were not successful.

Corte, Wolf, and Locke (1971) used food as a positive reinforcer for two profoundly retarded adolescents who had been institutionalized for at least ten years. SIB had occurred for at least four years. Subject One slapped his face repeatedly. Subject Two slapped her face, poked her eye, poked her tongue, and hit her face against the floor and chair. During a 15-minute session, the subjects were given candy for every 16 seconds without SIB. If a SIR was emitted, a 45-second period passed before another reinforcement. In the first phase the candy was given without food deprivation. In the second phase the candy was changed to a spoonful of thick malt, and lunch was withheld on the days of the experimental sessions. In the first phase SIB did not decrease for Subject One, but decreased to zero during the second phase with food deprivation. Subject Two did not show any change in SIB under either condition. The researchers questioned the practicality of this procedure, which was successful for only one subject under food deprivation.

Peterson and Peterson (1968) worked with an eight-year-old, nonverbal, ambulatory boy who had been placed in an institution for two years because he was unmanageable at home. The subject displayed no SIB while on the bed wrapped in a small quilt. When not in bed, the subject slapped the side of his head, hit his hand against his teeth, banged his forehead against his forearm, and struck his head and hands against furniture and walls. The sessions took place during lunchtime for 15 minutes. If a three- to five-second period of no SIR occurred, he was given one-quarter teaspoon of food. If a SIR occurred, the researcher took the food from the table and turned away from the subject for a period of ten seconds. If no SIR occurred during the ten seconds, the researcher turned back to the subject, said "good," and gave him a bite of food. The mean number of responses during this experimental period was 14.2 SIRs per minute. The mean number of responses before treatment was 26.6 SIRs per minute.

A second procedure was introduced in which the subject was to walk across the room and sit in a chair when a SIR occurred. If a SIR did not occur, he was given a bite of food. If a SIR did occur, he was instructed to walk back across the room and sit in a chair. During this procedure, the response rate dropped to below ten responses per session for six sessions and then became variable, reaching a high of 26 responses per minute before stabilizing to less than five responses per minute at session 54. The researchers stated the SIB was extinguished. The last recording of their total study was session 80. There were five sessions of baseline and three sessions for a reversal period.

Saposnek and Watson (1974) eliminated SIB in a ten-year-old boy diagnosed as autistic and mentally retarded by using techniques for rage reduction. Head slapping was accompanied by screaming, kicking, and flailing of body parts, which the experimenters considered tantrum behavior or rage. The experimenters believed the rage could be confronted by physically restraining the child during the tantrum and by the subject's slapping the experimenter's hand, which would be incompatible with head slapping. In the procedure, the subject was held in the experimenter's lap. When the subject began to scream, kick, and flail, he was physically restrained by the experimenter, the hand was blocked as he attempted to slap his head, and the experimenter manually guided the child's hand to slap the experimenter's hand, saying, "Hit my hand." After the second treatment session, the child voluntarily hit the experimenter's hand instead of his own. The head slapping behavior was reduced significantly to permit active participation in recreation, concept formation, and language training programs. The experimenters analyzed the procedure as a positive reinforcement paradigm, believing the hand slapping was positively reinforcing to the child.

Brawley, Harris, Allen, Fleming, and Peterson (1969), in a reversal research design, used social reinforcement in the form of adult attention to reduce self-hitting in a seven-year-old autistic boy. The adult attention was defined as touching the child, talking to, going to, and assisting the child. The researchers reported an average of three percent rate of self-hitting in the second extinction period compared to an average of 15 percent in the baseline period. Previous attention given to the SIB was believed to have maintained the behavior. The positive reinforcement and a carefully sequenced program increased the subject's verbal and academic skills. The subject began to seek and give attention and affection to the staff. The increased appropriate use of learning materials was incompatible with self-hitting and other inappropriate behaviors.

Negative Reinforcement

Treatment based on the negative reinforcement hypothesis assumes that SIB is maintained by the avoidance of an aversive stimulus following SIB. Treatment would be planned based on the hypothesis that an individual has learned that an aversive stimulus will be withdrawn or can be avoided if he engages in SIB. To test this hypothesis, treatment should be planned so that demands are not withdrawn as long as the subject engages in SIB. Instead, demands, or whatever stimulus is considered to be the aversive stimulus, would be maintained as long as the subject engages in SIB, and the aversive stimulus would be removed when the subject is not engaged in SIB.

Carr, Newson, and Binkoff (1976) noted that a psychotic child showed high rates of SIB in a classroom which was considered a demand situation, but the child would abruptly stop SIB when the stimulus to terminate the class was given. Carr (1977) suggested restraints may also serve as a means of escaping demand situations. As long as the individual is in restraints, demands will not be made upon him. Carr questioned whether compulsive thoughts and hallucinations might also play a role in escape-motivated SIB.

A study by Cautela and Baron (1973) may add some credence to Carr's hypothesis. The subject was a 20-year-old male diagnosed as schizophrenic, who two years prior to treatment withdrew from college because he was failing and found college meaningless. The subject began rubbing his eyes, saying they irritated him. No organic reason for the irritation could be found. The subject then began jabbing at his eyes. The subject began receiving psychotherapy and was diagnosed as obsessive-compulsive. The subject was treated with a variety of drugs including Chloralhydrate, Thorazine, Artane, Elavil, Mellaril, Librium, Paraldehyde, and Stelazine. These drugs had little effect on the SIB, and he was put in arm restraints and his eyes were sewn shut to prevent damage. The subject then began biting his lip and bit off the lower lip tissue. The resultant scar tissue formation caused him to have only one-half mouth opening. The subject's SIB caused swelling and bleeding of his eyes and face, saliva dripped from his mouth, and he was usually shaking and jerking his body. It is possible that the demands placed upon him as a student motivated the SIB. A multi-faceted behavior therapy program of relaxation, thought-stopping, covert sensitization, making a contract, systematic desensitization, and reinforcement sampling proved successful. These techniques gradually aided the subject to accept demand situations.

Punishment

Electric shock contingent upon SIB has been reported to be the most effective means of reducing or extinguishing SIB in the shortest length of time. Lovaas and Simmons (1969) used punishment procedures on an eight-year-old severely retarded boy who had SIB since two years of age. The subject's fists and knuckles were used to bang the temple and forehead. The parents had been partially successful in teaching the subject behaviors which were incompatible with SIB, such as holding objects in his hand. However, the subject gradually became increasingly uncontrollable and a decision was made to institutionalize him. The subject was in restraints for six months prior to the study. If restraints were removed, he would refuse to eat. The subject had been treated by extinction, but the results had not generalized to the experimental room. A second shock was given to the subject by a one-foot-long, hand-held inductorium. The shock was delivered from five 1.5-volt flashlight batteries with spikes as high as 1,400 volts at 50,000 ohms resistance. The shock was reported to be painful to the researcher and was compared to a dentist drilling on an unanesthetized tooth. Twelve shocks were given to the subject to gain control of the SIB. In future shocks, it was noticed that the subject was able to discriminate among researchers. Two other researchers administered shock, which brought about generalization. The behavior also lacked generalization across situations. Additional shock in other situations was needed to prevent SIB in other rooms.

Young and Wincz (1974) examined three treatment variables: the effect of reinforcing a behavior which is compatible with head banging, a behavior which is incompatible with head banging, and electric shock. The subject was a 21-year-old profoundly retarded girl who had been hospitalized continuously for 18 years. In order to prevent her from banging her head against the bed rails and hitting her head with her fists, she was restrained in bed. Ice cream was used to reinforce each eye contact, a compatible behavior, and hands on the wheels of wheelchair, a behavior incompatible with head banging. Baseline was obtained in the first phase. A return to baseline phase followed the second phase. The hands on wheels was the fourth phase. The fifth phase was the administration of electric shock plus reinforcement of incompatible behavior. The results showed the compatible behavior increased but did not reduce SIB. The reinforcement of incompatible behavior increased the incompatible behavior but did not reduce SIB. The generalization of behavior after shock was not reported.

Tate (1972) reported on a case study in which the goal was to reduce the frequency of SIB, so the subject could live in the institution without being restrained, drugged, or protected by padding. The limited time the researcher had and the roughly 14-year history of the behavior caused the researcher to focus on reducing the SIB, rather than to be concerned with a rigorous scientific study. The subject was an 18½-year-old female who had been restrained in bed for seven and one-half years. The subject was taken out of bed once a day to be bathed. Bathing the subject required six attendants to prevent self-injury. Multiple treatment procedures were used with the notion that a variety of procedures would maximize the chances of reducing the self-injury. No evidence was obtained on the effectiveness of the multiple techniques or of any single technique used. The goal of reducing self-injury to permit the subject to live in the institution free of restraints was achieved for a time. The behavior returned some time between seven months and three years after therapy due to undetermined causes. Tate found shock to be the most efficient procedure among the multiple types used. Tate concluded that a combination of punishment (response-contingent shock) and negative reinforcement (termination of shock) on cessation of responding may be highly effective in controlling self-injury.

The controlling effects of punishment are still subject to question. Aronfreed and Reber (1965) studied punishment effects on children of middle-class and working-class parents. Middle-class children showed more of a corresponding orientation toward internal monitors in control of behavior, and working-class children showed more of a corresponding orientation toward external monitors. A conclusion the researchers made from the study was that punishment of an act at its initiation is more effective than punishment at its completion. The factors mediating punishment effects may differ from individual to individual, since Romanczyck and Goren (1975) showed a much lower rate of SIB when shock was applied for hits making physical contact compared to shock applied prior to hits making physical contact.

Birnbrauer (1968) used contingent electric shock to eliminate infrequent and unpredictable biting and destructive acts of a 14-year-old, profoundly retarded subject. The subject had previously been treated by regression therapy, emotional feeding, electro-convulsive therapy, drugs, and restraints. The initial effects of shock punishment were dramatically positive. The author cautions researchers on the limitations of punishment, however, because of the highly discriminative nature of its effects. Lasting therapeutic effects were not achieved. The subject in this study was not self-injurious, but the study emphasized the difficulty in generalization of the effects of punishment reported in the earlier studies using punishment.

Because of the highly discriminative abilities of subjects under shock punishment treatment, Buchar and King (1971) stated that the punishment should be associated with natural environmental contingencies in which the unwanted behavior is to be suppressed. After a period of receiving shock punishment treatment, some children learn to terminate the unwanted behavior at the verbal signal, "No!" which had been paired with shock during the treatment.

Obtaining generalization of the effects of electric shock has been one of the problems noted by researchers advocating the use of shock to reduce SIB. Ethical considerations prevent general distribution of shock prods to staff with which to provide electric shock when subjects engage in SIB in different settings. Tanner and Zeiler (1975) studied the effect of using aromatic ammonia as the aversive stimulus to reduce SIB. The ammonia capsules were relatively safe, inexpensive, and easily concealed, so a patient would have difficulty discriminating the staff member who was to provide the aversive stimulus. The procedure was effective. Long-term follow-up was not possible due to the patient's being transferred to another institution. Some negative effects were that it would be difficult to physically place the capsule effectively near a strong, agile, and mobile patient; the ammonia fumes irritated the staff person; and the odor remained for some time on the person's finger. Scabs were reported to occur on the patient's nose; however, the researchers reported that it was not known whether the scabs were due to the ammonia capsule's coming in contact with the subject's nose or whether they were due to the subject's upper respiratory infection.

Since punishment has been most frequently reported as being most effective to reduce SIB, researchers have studied less aversive forms of punishment. Kelly and Drabman (1977) used a form of over-correction as a form of punishment for a three-year-old, blind male who poked his eye. The over-correction procedure was carried out by the teacher, who lowered and raised the subject's arm 12 times to simulate an eye poke each time the subject touched his eye with his hand. After a ten-minute over-correction period, the subject was allowed to play with other children and toys for 20 minutes. During the play time, eye pokes were ignored. Initially there was a response burst in which the number of eye poking responses rose above the baseline rate. Following the initial rise in response rate, the eye poking gradually declined until it reached near zero. The mean response rate was 3.3 percent during treatment, compared to the mean of 23.4 percent during baseline.

Differential Reinforcement of Alternative Behavior
In the differential reinforcement of alternative behavior, the experimenter ignored the SIB and reinforced the subject for engaging in incompatible, alternative, or socially more acceptable behavior (Baumeister and Rollings, 1976). Reinforcement for behaviors which are incompatible with the SIB has been reported to have varying degrees of success in reducing SIB (Frankel, Moss, Schofield and Simmons, 1976; Frankel and Simmons, 1976). The incompatible behaviors being taught and reinforced range from static position to active, socially appropriate and pleasure-producing movements.

Lovaas et al. (1965) taught a nine-year-old subject to clap and rock with the rhythm of the music and to bar-press. These behaviors, which were incompatible with the subject's SIB, reduced the SIB. Saposnek and Watson (1974) taught a ten-year-old subject to slap the experimenter's hand instead of the subject's hand. Reinforcing hand slapping reduced the SIB significantly and enabled the subject to participate in educational and recreational activities.

Myers and Diebert (1971) reinforced a seven-year-old subject if his hands were held at the side of his body. SIB was reduced sufficiently so that the subject was able to be sent home, but his behavior deteriorated at home. The subject was reinstitutionalized and SIB was again reduced using the same procedure. The new behavior did not generalize to other situations.

Young and Wincze (1974) reinforced a 21-year-old for holding his hands on the wheelchair. The incompatible behavior did not reduce the SIB. Measel and

Alfieri (1976) studied the effect of reinforcing peg placement in a pegboard in a 14-year-old subject. The reinforcers, which included manual guidance, verbal praise, and pats on the back, did not have a positive effect on the SIB.

Some behavioral scientists (Baumeister and Rollings, 1976) refer to these procedures as differential reinforcement of other behaviors. The other behaviors may include the absence of SIB. In this procedure, a reinforcement was delivered contingent on a specified time interval of nonoccurrence of SIB. Each occurrence of SIB reset this interval.

Allen and Harris (1966) reinforced all desirable behaviors in a five-year-old subject and withheld reinforcement for SIB of scratching the face, neck, and body. Social approval, candy, and presentation of dolls served as reinforcers. The SIB was reduced within a six-month period, resulting in the disappearance of scabs and open sores.

Bites of food were used to reinforce periods of any behavior other than SIB in two adolescent subjects studied by Corte, Wolf, and Locke (1971). The procedure was effective with one subject under mild food deprivation but was not effective for either of the two subjects when under no food deprivation.

Some studies have reported success using a combination of procedures. Measel and Alfieri (1976) found reinforcement of incompatible behavior ineffective in reducing SIB in a 14-year-old subject. The researchers chose to combine the over-correction regimen used by Azrin, Kaplan, and Foxx (1973) in eliminating self-stimulating behaviors with reinforcement of incompatible behavior to study the effect on SIB. The over-correction regimen required the subject to maintain both arms in three successive positions for 30 seconds in each position. The subject was expected to position the arms in these positions upon corresponding verbal cues of "hands up," "hands out," and "hands down." If there was no response by three seconds, the hands were positioned by the experimenter by manual guidance. The researchers found that the reinforcement, combined with a verbal reprimand for the first SIB and a two-minute over-correction following a second SIB within a predetermined interval of time, was more effective than reinforcement alone. The SIB was controlled by verbal reprimand alone by the ninth session. Four months following the termination of treatment, the subject was observed in a classroom for random 15-minute periods during four hours in the morning. No SIB was observed for six observation days.

A second study by Measel and Alfieri (1976) with a second 16-year-old subject using a head movement over-correction regimen resulted in an increase in SIB. The researchers discontinued the study following the seventh session after four previous sessions showed a rapid increase in SIB. The researchers concluded that the over-correction regimen was probably reinforcing the SIB.

Ragain and Anson (1976) used bites of the evening meal to reinforce five-second intervals without SIB. The subject was a 14-year-old who continuously scratched her shoulder and back and banged her head. Extinction and noncontingent reinforcement were also used in this study. As the SIB came under stimulus control, the interval was increased gradually to 30-second intervals. Although SIB was not totally eliminated, the study showed that SIB could be placed under stimulus control.

An adaptation of the over-correction hand control regimen (Azrin et al., 1973) was used by deCatanzaro and Baldwin (1978) to reduce head hitting by an eight-year-old and a 12-year-old subject. Upon a head hitting response, the experimenter held the wrist of the subject and gently pumped it up and down. This procedure resulted in a decrease in head hitting. The procedure was combined with differential reinforcement of other behaviors. The reinforcers were pats on the back and gentle rocking movements applied to the subject's wheelchair. The combined procedure resulted in a near zero SIR rate. Both subjects had been in restraints, which were gradually removed until all physical restraints were able to be removed. The subjects were able to be included in programs in which the hands could be used in constructive activities.

Self-injurious air swallowing (aerophagia) in two profoundly mentally retarded individuals was treated by a contingent coactive mouth covering procedure (Holburn and Dougher, 1985). Air swallowing decreased in one client but increased in the other. A variation of the procedure was used with the client who showed increased aerophagia. Each time the client touched the experimenter's hand, which was on the table in front of the client, she received the three seconds of hand placement over her mouth. The procedure reduced aerophagia, but complete suppression did not occur (Holburn and Dougher, 1986).

Repp and Deitz (1974) studied the effect of differential reinforcement of other behaviors, plus a mild verbal reprimand versus a mild verbal reprimand alone. The subject was a ten-year-old, institutionalized girl who scratched her face. M & M candy was used as the reinforcer and given at fixed intervals contingent on nonoccurrence of SIB during that interval. There was a significant reduction in SIB with the combination of differential reinforcement of other behaviors and mild, verbal reprimand. The mild, verbal reprimand alone did not decrease SIB. The authors stated the difficulty in determining the effect of differential reinforcement of other behaviors because of its use with other procedures.

Baumeister and Rollings (1976) noted that most studies using differential reinforcement of other behaviors were confounded by the use of many variables, making it difficult to determine the effect of differential reinforcement of other behaviors alone. Studies of differential reinforcement of other behaviors have established that under some circumstances the SIB can be brought under temporary control.

Restraining the individual has been the most common form of treatment for SIB. Restraints have prevented the individual from physically self-injuring while the restraint was securely on the individual. Objections to restraints have been that restraints masked the SIB as well as other behaviors. The restrained individual was not able to participate in motor activities. Prolonged periods in restraints have resulted in irreversible physical deformities such as joint contractions and demineralization of bones. Frequently, when restraints were removed even for basic care such as bathing and dressing, there were increased bursts of SIB. The advantages of the restraints have been that they were easily applied and economical. However, the problems apparent raised ethical considerations and have shown restraints to be an aversive and undesirable form of treatment (Azrin et al., 1975; Picker et al., 1979).

Psychodynamic treatment has not been effective in reducing SIB. The reported cases of psychodynamic treatment were used in combination with other methods (Carr, 1977; Crabtree, 1967). Chemotherapy has had questionable value in treatment of SIB (Peterson and Peterson, 1968; Picker et al., 1979). Corbett (1975) has stated that neurosurgical intervention cannot be considered a feasible treatment at the present time. According to Carr (1977), the sensory stimulation theory has merit but has not been adequately tested. The treatments based on learning theory have resulted in reduction and extinction of SIB for some individuals for short periods (Carr, 1977; Picker et al., 1979; Smolev, 1971). Treatment procedures using extinction, punishment, and other aversive methods have raised sufficient ethical questions to make them undesirable

methods of treatment. Other behavior modification techniques which have reported success have been based on single cases in which treatment was conducted over a short period of time and follow-up reports were not made to report the lasting effects (Azrin et al., 1975). Picker et al. (1979) reported that of over 60 studies reviewed in 1978, most were methodologically unsophisticated case studies.

In Corbett's (1975) review of studies on SIB, noncontingent stimulation for treating stereotyped behaviors was felt to be relevant to the study of SIB. A conclusion was made after a review of the studies that a generally enriched environment which is not overstimulating will tend to reduce stereotyped behavior in the retarded. A further conclusion was made that there is little evidence for any beneficial effect of noncontingent stimulation on severe SIB, and that ". . . injudicious and unplanned stimulation may in fact aggravate matters" (p. 86).

Noncontingent stimulation studies which used visual, auditory, and manipulative objects were reviewed by Corbett (1975). Case studies in which noncontingent somatosensory stimulation is normally provided during the healthy parent-infant bonding period are infrequently reported (Bright et al., 1981; Lemke, 1974; Wells and Smith, 1983).

Most of the reported treatment has been based on learning theories. Treatment techniques reported to be successful in reducing SIB have not gained widespread use because of legal and ethical concerns (Lovaas and Simmons, 1969; Smolev, 1971) or because of the impracticality of implementing the procedure (Tate and Baroff, 1966). Many reportedly successful techniques have been successful only in the research setting, and thus have questionable value.

Chapter III

THE EFFECT OF TACTILE STIMULATION ON SELF-INJURIOUS BEHAVIOR

Self-injurious behavior (SIB) poses a difficult management problem. It appears that variables other than the specific SIB are operating simultaneously in some self-injurious individuals, since techniques which successfully extinguish SIB in some individuals have not proven successful with others.

Successful results in the reduction of SIB have been reported using contingent sensory stimulation such as olfactory in the form of aromatic ammonia (Baumeister and Baumeister, 1978); tactile in the form of water mist to the face (Dorsey et al., 1980); tactile and kinesthetic by handling objects (Mantione, 1977); tactile, olfactory, and gustatory in the form of food (Peterson and Peterson, 1968); and visual and auditory in the form of smiles and verbal praise (Lovaas et al., 1965).

Noncontingent sensory stimulation has been suggested as a method to reduce SIB based on the presumption that certain levels of somatosensory stimulation, primarily tactile, vestibular, and kinesthetic, are necessary or desirable for human beings. If so, when somatosensory stimulation is inadequate, the individual may engage in SIB as a form of self-stimulation, simply to provide somatosensory input (Fisher, 1974; Baumeister and Foreman, 1973; Montagu, 1971; Cleland and Clark, 1966; Berkson and Mason, 1963; Lourie, 1949). By providing appropriate stimulation, SIB may be reduced, since somatosensory input may now be adequate. Case studies in which somatosensory stimulation plus social stimulation proved successful, reported by Bright, Bittick, and Fleeman (1981); Lemke (1974); and Wells and Smith (1983), give some credence to this possibility.

It seemed worthwhile to study the effect of noncontingent sensory stimulation more systematically and with a larger population. Isolating one form of sensory stimulation is difficult, however, an attempt was made to emphasize tactile stimulation administered to specific areas of the body in predetermined quantity and duration. If successful, the procedure could be an effective method for generic, direct-care staff to reduce SIB in the severely and profoundly retarded, non-ambulatory subjects.

Methodology

The subjects were eight institutionalized, nonambulatory, nonverbal subjects, between 16.5 and 18.5 years old, who were displaying SIB, and were diagnosed as mentally retarded based on IQ scores derived from the Slosson Intelligence Tests administered by staff psychologists. The severity of the SIB for each subject was such that the cottage staff considered it difficult to prevent self-injury or to handle the individual except by restricting movement, and thus referred the subject for treatment. One group of four subjects was selected from each of two cottages. The description of the subjects in the two groups are summarized in Table 1.

All eight subjects directed self-injury to their head and mouth, and used their hand to either injure body parts or injure parts of the hand itself. Six of the eight subjects hit, scratched, or rubbed their head. Three subjects rubbed, pressed, or poked their eyes. Four subjects hit or scratched their ears. Six subjects bit their fingers or thumb.

The study was conducted at a state facility in New Jersey, a 1,000-bed, residential institution for the mentally retarded. The annual survey revealed residents ranged in age from 6 to 73 years, with a mean of 25 years. Ninety-two percent were classified as severely and profoundly retarded, and 31 percent were self-injurious.

The institution had 18 one-floor residential cottages. Each cottage had sleeping, bathing, and day activity areas. An office and one or two rooms for educational

Table 1

Description of Subjects

Group Subject	Sex	CA	IQ	Medical Condition	Current Restraints	Previous Treatment	SIRs*
A-1	M	17.42	7	Downs Syndrome	Helmet Cervical Collar	Behavior Mod.** Restraints	Hits head, throat, jaw, ear, chest, stomach, knee, leg, arm; pokes eye; bites finger; scratches head.
A-2	M	16.66	6	Blind Scoliosis Oral Defect	Helmet	Behavior Mod.** Restraints	Rubs and pokes eye; bites finger; hits head, shoulder, ear, cheek, foot; bangs elbow, head against wall.
A-3	M	17.59	3	Blind	Helmet	Behavior Mod.**	Presses eye, cheeks; bites fingers, hand; pinches and pulls skin; scratches arm; hits head, ears, nose, cheek, jaw, chest, leg.
A-4	M	17.25	3	Blind			Scratches head, nose; rubs head.
	x̄	= 17.23					
B-1	F	18.50	3	Blind	Helmet Mittens		Bangs head; pulls hair.
B-2	M	17.66	2	Spastic Quadriplegia Hydrocephalus Blind Scoliosis Hips Dislocated	Thumb Splint	Restraints	Sucks, bites thumb.
B-3	F	16.50	7	Microcephalic Seizures	Elbow Restraints Cervical Collar Mittens	Restraints	Rubs, scratches head; bites thumb, thenar prominence, wrist; digs ear, nose; pushes whole hand in mouth, induces vomiting.
B-4	M	18.50	2	Spastic Quadriplegia Scoliosis Dislocated Left Hip Seizures			Bites, sucks thumb.
	x̄	= 17.79					

*See Table 2 **Description of Behavior Modification
Twenty-minute sessions were conducted by a psychology department technician (trainer). If a helmet was worn, it was removed. Following 30 seconds without injury, an object was presented to the subject. The trainer verbally praised the subject during noninjury. If the subject self-injured, the trainer said firmly, "No (e.g., *hitting*) (*subject's name*)," while holding the subject's hands down for 30 seconds. After 30 seconds, the trainer released the hands and repeated the procedure by presenting the object and speaking to the subject.

programs and conferences were part of each cottage. All cottages were kept locked.

In Group A's cottage, most residents spent waking hours in their wheelchairs or carts, or on the floor in a large room. In Group B's cottage, residents spent waking hours in their beds, carts, or wheelchairs in their rooms or in wheelchairs or carts in the hallway.

To eliminate the usual random auditory, visual, and social stimuli, an available quiet area was used for the baseline and stimulation sessions. Sessions for Group A were held in a hallway and for Group B in a corner of the conference room. A 4' × 8' mat was placed on the floor, and the subject was wheeled to the mat and placed seated or supine on the mat. The therapist sat on the mat facing the subject. The recorder sat in a chair against the opposite wall from the mat for Group A and an equal distance away for Group B. Random announcements over the loudspeaker were the only unexpected stimuli.

Staff Training
Two certified occupational therapy assistants served as therapists, while two registered occupational therapists served as recorders. They were trained in four sessions prior to the study. The recorders were instructed how to complete a developmental checklist (including skills in gross- and fine-motor, feeding, dressing, toileting, bathing, communication, and play) and a SIB profile (compiled for each subject to determine areas of the body injured). The definition of SIB as used in this study was discussed, and precise definitions of each self-injurious response (SIR) targeted for each subject were clarified. A list was provided which specified the types of SIRs, with the duration or rate required for a single response to be recorded.

Single events of a bang, bite, hit, pinch, poke, pull, and scratch were recorded as a single response. Long durations of the above were recorded as a single response for each continuous second.

Tally sheets listing all of the identified SIRs for each subject were prepared following completion of the SIB profile. The recorders observed each session and continuously recorded each response on the tally sheet. Hand counters were available for use during bursts of rapid responses. A large wall clock with second hand was in the area; however, recorders were instructed to silently count "1001" as one second.

In general, *self-injurious behavior* (SIB) was defined as any self-inflicted physical contact to the body which results in observable physical injury or change which interferes with the normal growth and development of the individual. A *self-injurious response* (SIR) was defined as a single unit of SIB. Examples of SIRs in the study were: *Hitting*—this was defined as a series of hits to a body part which takes place during a one-second period of time; *Poking*—this was defined as a sudden jabbing movement to a body part with one or more digits; *Biting*—this was defined as clamping a body part between the teeth. SIR definitions and measurement were tailored to the individual patterns of each subject (see Tables 1 and 2). Observer reliability above .90 (smaller/larger) was established prior to the beginning of the baseline recording with target residents not in this study.

A treatment manual (see Appendix) with detailed written instructions and illustrations of the body parts to be given tactile stimulation was given to each recorder and therapist. A videotape was shown in which the researcher demonstrated on a normal person the sequence of tactile stimulation. The direction of the movements, the parts of the therapist's hands to be

used, and the number of times to stimulate a particular area were demonstrated.

Procedure
Baseline: Each group of subjects was assigned a recorder who obtained baseline data. The length of baseline period was predetermined for each subject. A separate, independent observer recorded two reliability checks during the baseline period.

During each baseline session, the therapist removed all restraints from the subject and sat on the mat with the subject during a 30-minute session. The recorder sat as described earlier and recorded each SIR. The total number of SIRs was plotted on a graph after each session. If the SIRs had the potential to cause serious injury if left unrestrained according to prior information from the medical staff, the restraints were to be reapplied. Subject B3's sessions were frequently terminated early, due to induced vomiting. This subject averaged 14.4-minute sessions in baseline and 15-minute sessions in treatment. For this subject only, the number of SIRs was extrapolated for the amount of time remaining in the session. All other subjects completed all sessions. Subjects number 1 in both groups had a 5-day baseline, subjects number 2 in both groups had an 8-day baseline, subjects number 3 in both groups had an 11-day baseline, and subjects number 4 in both groups had a 14-day baseline.

Treatment: SIRs were counted and recorded during the treatment sessions, as in the baseline data collecting and recording. Reliability checks were made twice for

Table 2
*Definitions of SIRs

Bang:	Striking a body part against an immovable surface, resulting in inflammation or elevation of the surface of the body.
Bite:	Clamping a body part between the teeth.
Hit:	Striking a body part with closed or open hand.
Pinch:	Sudden squeeze and release of a body part between thumb and finger(s).
Poke:	Sudden jabbing movement to a body part with one or more digits.
Scratch:	Moving one or more fingernails against the skin, causing an inflamed line or tear in the skin.
Pull:	Sustained holding of a body part between thumb and fingers and pulling away from body.
Press:	Sustained pressure against a body part with one or more fingers, causing displacement of the body part.
Rub:	Sustained moving pressure against a body part by another body part, causing inflammation.
Suck:	Sustained pressure on a body part with tongue, mouth, and lips, causing inflammation and swelling.
Induce Vomit:	Open or closed hand placed into back of mouth, causing food and gastric juices to surface.

*See Table 1

Table 3

Sequence and Nature of Stimulation in Treatment Sessions

Sequence	Body Part	Number of Times	Duration Each Time
1. Stroke lateral edge of eyes to hairline bilaterally		3	1 sec
2. Stroke lateral edge of lips to temple bilaterally		3	1 sec
3. Stroke lateral edge of lips to base of earlobe bilaterally		3	1 sec
4. Stroke base of earlobe to lateral edge of lips bilaterally		3	1 sec
5. Press above and below lips		8	1 sec
6. Stroke base of earlobe to collarbone bilaterally		3	1 sec
7. Stroke chin to collarbone		1	3 sec
8. Stroke with palms from shoulder to elbow bilaterally		5	3 sec
9. Stroke each finger from base to tip		1	3 sec
10. Squeeze each finger repeatedly from base to tip		6 (1 sec each squeeze; 6 squeezes each finger)	1 sec
11. Stroke each forearm from wrist to elbow		5	3 sec
12. Squeeze each forearm repeatedly		5	2 sec
13. Brief break during which the therapist guided subject in functional activity (e.g., clapping, handling object)			5 min
14. Squeeze each leg repeatedly, ankle to knee		10	2 sec
15. Stroke sole of foot, toes to heel		3	3 sec
16. Stroke sides of each toe simultaneously		1	2 sec
17. Squeeze each toe repeatedly from base to tip		3 (1 sec each squeeze; 3 squeezes each toe)	1 sec
18. Brief break during which the therapist guided subject in functional activity (e.g., pushing feet against stable surface, weight bearing, if possible)			5 min

each subject during the treatment phase. The first check was made during the first five days of treatment. The second check was made randomly during the remainder of the treatment phase.

One therapist was assigned to each group of subjects. Treatment sessions were 30 minutes long and were held each morning Monday through Friday.

The treatment consisted of tactile stimulation applied to the face, neck, shoulders, upper extremities, and on the lower extremities from the knees to the toes. The therapists were asked not to verbalize except to say "Hello (name of subject)" at the beginning of the session and "Good-bye (name of subject)" at the end of the session. If the subject was known to be assaultive to others as well as self-injurious, the usual disciplinary measures used by the cottage staff were maintained during the treatment session.

Tactile stimulation was provided by the tips of the index and middle fingers of the hand(s), and occasionally (noted in Table 3) with the palms of the hands. It was gentle, but firm enough to temporarily indent the skin. The stimulation was precisely specified in terms of location and duration, in order to avoid any possible contingent use of stimulation. Therapists did not restrain or prevent SIRs during treatment. The locations, times, and sequence of stimulation are shown in Table 3.

Reliability was calculated by the formula smaller divided by larger. The reliability measures for baseline and treatment ranged from .90 to 1.00. The mean reliability measure for Group A was .99 and for Group B was .98.

Results

Figures 1 and 2 show the SIR rates during the baseline and treatment phases for Groups A and B, respectively. In Group A, SIR rates decreased markedly for each subject. Subject 1 decreased from an average of 199.2 instances in baseline to 34.5 in treatment; subject 2 decreased from 144.5 instances to 37.0; subject 3, from 212.0 to 37.8; and subject 4, from 14.7 to 5.2. Similar results were shown for Group B, thus replicating the effects across therapists and subjects. In this group, subject 1 went from 32.6 instances to 5.6; subject 2, from 9.9 to 4.3; subject 3, from 245.0 to 75.9; and subject 4, from 12.6 to 9.3.

The percentage decreases these numbers represent are fairly large. Subject A1 showed an 82.7% decrease in SIR rate from the baseline to the treatment phase; subject A2 showed a 74.4% decrease; subject A3, an 82.1% decrease; and subject A4, a 64.6% decrease. Similar effects occurred in Group B. Subject B1 showed an 82.8% decrease in SIR rate from the baseline phase to

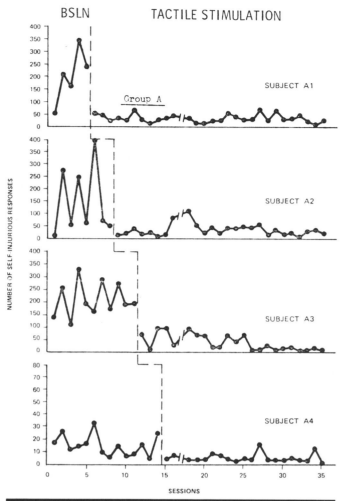

Figure 1

Self-injurious responses for group A during baseline and tactile stimulation sessions.

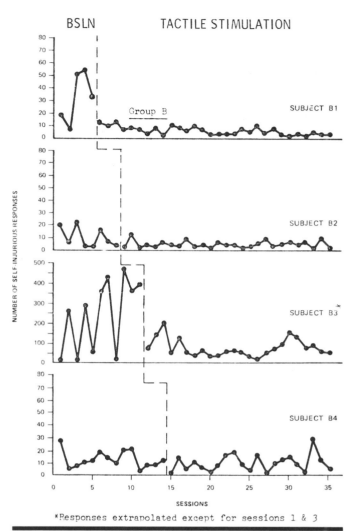

Figure 2

Self-injurious responses for group B during baseline and tactile stimulation sessions.

the treatment phase; subject B2 showed a 56.8% decrease; subject B3, a 69.1% decrease; and subject B4, a 26.2% decrease.

Treatment effects seemed greatest for the subjects with the highest initial rates of SIR (A1, A2, A3, B1, B3), those who injured more areas of the body, and those who used more variety in the method of self-injury (A1, A2, A3, B3). Stable reductions in SIR were seen in all subjects, however.

A number of related effects were also anecdotally reported. Comments were recorded by the observers on the tally sheets after each session. In both groups each subject with vision made more frequent eye contact with the therapist for increasing lengths of time. During the course of treatment, subjects changed from defensive and aggressive activities to passively accepting the treatment, and eventually actively trying to engage the therapist to provide the tactile stimulation. For example, subject A1 took the therapist's hand

and placed it on his body part to be stimulated. Subject A2 initially did not permit stimulation on the face but, as the treatment sessions continued, allowed the tactile stimulation. Cottage staff reported that subject A2 was generally less defensive around his eyes, nose and neck, noted during bathing and feeding. Subject A3 initially resisted treatment and tried to bite the therapist. The defensive and aggressive behaviors gradually disappeared in subject A3. Cottage staff reported increased vocalizations and decreased self-stimulating behaviors in all subjects. Following completion of the study, three subjects in Group A were able to begin self-help programs.

Discussion

Results suggest that noncontingent tactile stimulation decreased SIB in these non-ambulatory, nonverbal, profoundly retarded, institutionalized adolescents. Data from the two groups show that effects of the stimulation generalized across subjects, settings, and experimenters. The greater treatment effect seen for the subjects with the higher baseline rates of SIR and those who injured more areas of their body using a variety of methods to self-injure may be indicative of the self-stimulating effect of SIB for those subjects.

Tactile stimulation in the above studies provide an area for speculation about its effect on the SIB in those studies. Dorsey, Iwata, Reed, and Davis (1982) suggest that the combination of contingent protective equipment and access to sensory-stimulating toys may maintain levels of decreased SIB.

If noncontingent tactile stimulation can reduce SIB in institutionalized residents, there are additional benefits to consider: (1) The procedure requires minimal added expense, since additional equipment is not required. (2) Treatment can be incorporated into the existing daily bathing, feeding, play, and education routine. (3) Staff efforts would shift from application of restraints and separation from the resident to interaction and educational efforts. (4) Attitudes would change from fear of being responsible for the resident's SIB to that of helping the resident learn and develop. (5) The treatment procedure could be easily taught to direct-care staff.

Additional study using tactile stimulation is recommended because of the limitations of this study. This study is limited by the lack of data outside the treatment sessions and results of long-term effects. Institutional administrative concerns limited this study by time, location, and staff. The focus needed to be limited to short-term effects of tactile stimulation provided outside the area where the subjects routinely spent the day.

Additional research using tactile stimulation noncontingently would help clarify its effect on subjects with SIB. In the noncontingent stimulation studies reviewed by Corbett (1975), the stimulation affected visual and auditory receptors rather than the somatosensory receptors, which are affected by tactile stimulation. In this study, the changes in the quality of responses anecdotally reported suggest that even the minimal amount of purposeful activity and play facilitated in the treatment sessions helped to maintain the reduced level of SIB.

Future studies using noncontingent tactile stimulation should identify any neurological reflexive responses of potential subjects. Such subjects may not respond to the currently described stimulation, since other types of treatment may be needed for the neurological condition. Subjects B2 and B4 in this study were diagnosed as spastic quadriplegic. Subject B4 had a seizure disorder. It is speculated that the reflexive activity accounted for the variable responses seen in these two subjects.

In summary, this study suggests that tactile stimulation given noncontingently to individuals with SIB may satisfy some of their needs for somatosensory stimulation and reduce SIB. Replication of the study is needed to identify those individuals for which this stimulation is most effective. The treatment is an economical, safe, and easily administered procedure.

Chapter IV

A SENSORIMOTOR TREATMENT PROGRAM

The etiology of self-injurious behavior (SIB) is unknown. The previous chapter reviewed the author's research on the effect of tactile stimulation on SIB. The research suggests that tactile stimulation reduced SIB significantly for six of eight individuals.

In many situations, it is not possible to replicate reported successful programs. Reported programs are not appropriate for all individuals with SIB. Still, parents, therapists, and teachers are responsible for the daily management of the self-injurious individual. For these individuals, suggestions are given on how to implement a practical sensorimotor program aimed at providing stimulation and training in those daily living skills the patient is capable of learning.

Assumptions

The treatment program is based on the following assumptions: 1) The individual needs basic stimulation to the body and mind. This stimulation needs to be provided for the individual if he or she is limited in mobility. In some cases when the person is capable of self-initiated stimulation, the person needs direction as to the optimal type and amount of stimulation. 2) The individual needs to have some sense of control over his or her own body in order to affect survival, self-care, or the state of well-being. 3) The individual needs to interact with environmental forces, objects, and people in order to maintain a state of physical and mental well-being. Such interaction is needed for the person to develop and to grow. 4) For some individuals the beginning of SIB may be an attempt to communicate any of the above needs.

An assumption is also made that repetitive, self-stimulating behaviors are part of a range of behaviors that can lead to SIB when proper kinds and amounts of stimulation are unavailable to the person.

It is possible for anyone to have an irritant or itch occur in the eye or ear, on the scalp, or on other parts of the body. Normally, people automatically rub, scratch, or slap the area of the irritant or itch to counteract the undesired feeling.

It is possible for anyone to have a headache, earache, toothache or joint or muscle pain. This type of pain may more likely occur in people who are maintained in static positions for long periods, in those who have infrequent dental examinations and inadequate oral care, and in those who are given minimal physical attention. Anyone who is verbal and alert can communicate a need for attention. An individual who is nonverbal or mentally retarded has difficulty communicating about any pain or discomfort.

If attention is unavailable and the pain or discomfort is not removed, the individual may try to rub, slap, scratch, or try other physical means to eliminate the pain or discomfort. The same types of behavior may be tried by an individual to produce stimulation to the body.

In the process of trying to eliminate pain or discomfort or in trying to generate stimulation to the body, a desired response may occur by chance. The response may be given by a person, or the response may be a bodily feeling that is more desirable than the prior feeling caused by pain, discomfort, or lack of stimulation.

The individual may learn that the self-stimulating or self-injurious behavior results in verbal attention, physical handling, movement, being left alone, or any number of desired responses. The responses, which may be viewed as negative or positive by the individual, may be repeated. The cycle becomes established. The self-stimulating or self-injurious individual thus learns how to use SIB to control the environment, including people, to serve his or her own needs. The behavior which may not have been self-injurious in the beginning now can be labelled SIB by observers and caretakers, and their attitudes and behaviors can reinforce continued behavior by the individual. These are only assumptions, and they have not been researched by this author.

For simplicity, in the rest of this chapter the word patient will be used to refer to the individual with SIB.

Program Implementation

It is important for all persons concerned with the patient to understand as much as possible about the treatment program being planned. Many practical issues need to be agreed upon by all persons concerned. These issues include, but may not be limited to, those of space, time, expectations, outcomes, and future plans. The following kinds of questions should be answered. Where will the treatment take place? If the treatment is to be given in the patient's ward, classroom or therapy room, will the treatment interfere with other educational or therapy activities scheduled for the same time? How much time can be devoted to treatment of SIB? SIB is frequently considered of low priority. How many days or months are staff and administrators willing to allocate for this program? What changes in the patient will be acceptable to staff and administrators as signs that the patient has improved? Will improvement in the patient mean that other patients will be started on similar intensive treatment, or is the initial treatment program a trial-only program? If other patients are to be treated, can other staff be assigned to continue with certain aspects of the treatment if they are given supervision by the primary therapist?

A clear understanding of the above issues and other issues unique to the specific situation will help prevent false expectations, disappointments, and poorly conducted programs. Future plans for program continuation may prevent regression in the patient should improvement occur.

In most situations, a referral for therapy for the patient with SIB will not be routinely made. The therapist who desires implementing a treatment program will most likely need to elicit a referral. This will entail orientation of those persons directly involved in the care and education of the patient about various treatment methods, and the reason the therapist selected to use the sensorimotor approach.

An appropriate orientation to the treatment program for other staff members and for administrators is essential for the support of the program. After the preliminary orientation, administrative approval, and a referral to treat the patient have been obtained, other written permission-to-treat forms and letters should be obtained.

Permission to Treat

A written consent to evaluate and treat the patient should be secured from parents or guardians of the patient. This is particularly important since the patient behavior is one which can cause serious injury to the patient or to others if the patient is aggressive as well as self-injurious. When requesting permission, explain the possible range of patient reactions and outcomes.

It is possible that increased SIB may result when each new procedure is introduced. Understanding that the increased SIB is an expected reaction will prevent negative reactions from those expecting immediate, dramatic decrease in SIB. By the time a decision to terminate treatment is reached, it is possible that the patient will show no significant change in SIB, or a measurable reduction in SIB may result, or the SIB may be more intense, or SIB may be extinguished. There are so many unknown factors influencing SIB that no firm statement about outcome can be made. In most cases, improved behavior is seen.

If the patient is in or associated with a residential or educational facility, a committee may need to thoroughly review the treatment procedure and give approval before patient or guardian approval is requested. Possibly more than one committee will need to review and approve any new proposed treatment program. Depending on the particular situation, the committee members may be the only staff who need the initial orientation to the proposed treatment program.

As a precautionary measure, secure written permission to manually restrain the patient when necessary during treatment in order to prevent serious injury to the patient or, in the case of an aggressive patient, injury to the therapist. Most regulations prohibit application of physical restraints on patients without physician's orders.

Secure permission to review the patient's history and records. Background information is essential to effective treatment planning. Be cognizant of the laws related to confidentiality of personal information.

Permission to Photograph

Secure permission to film, videotape, and photograph the patient before, during, and following evaluation and treatment. Approval to do so should be in writing from the administrators of the facility and from the parents or guardians of the patient.

It is often difficult to accurately collect data and manage the treatment process with a patient when working alone. Most facilities have personnel available to videotape treatment procedures. In some instances, if the patient is not too active, it will be possible to set up the video camera and film independently. Review of videotapes will help analyze the behavior and treatment effects. Such documentation will help parents and others not directly involved in the actual treatment to understand the treatment process and to see patient gains, which may not be obvious from written documentation.

Permission to Conduct Research

If there is any plan to conduct research and report results, the intention must be stated before any treatment begins. The potential researcher should consult state and facility regulations on human research and obtain required approval.

Evaluation

An evaluation is made of the patient's SIB, the level of neurophysiological development, cognitive ability, psychosocial functioning, general adaptive functioning, and any specific skills and interests. Neurological, physical, and medical conditions and problems are noted since these will influence treatment methods used. Medical and physical problems can be overlooked because of the severe SIB and the focus on controlling the behavior. It is possible for medical, physical, and neurological conditions or medication to be the basis for the SIB.

Self-injurious Behavior

Before any treatment is given, observe the patient at various times of the day under various conditions in his or her usual setting. The amount of time spent in the initial observation and in gathering baseline data will depend upon the particular situation. The most important information to gather is the actual number of self-injurious responses in a given period of time over a given period of sessions. For treatment planning, it is important to look for and record other information about the SIB (see Appendix).

The following questions will alert the therapist to the SIB specific to the patient. What part of the body is injured most? Is one part injured more than another? Is there a set pattern to the way self-injury is accomplished, once started? For example, does the patient begin by hitting the left arm, then the right side of the face, then lean forward and hit the head on the floor? How is the self-injury accomplished? Does the patient slap, hit with a closed fist, poke, scratch, bite, or bang the body part against the floor or other hard surface?

What part of the body is used to accomplish the injury? Is the patient aggressive toward others? What behavior is manifest? How is the aggressive behavior accomplished? What conditions elicit aggressive behavior? If the patient is aggressive toward others, are there conditions under which the patient is not aggressive toward a particular person or persons? Be as descriptive as possible in recording answers to these and other questions. A clear, detailed description of the patient behavior prior to treatment will help analyze changes in the behavior.

Record the number of self-injurious responses in a given number of minutes in the patient's normal setting for three to five days. Record data at the same time each day. If possible, have a second person independently record data at the same time to establish reliability for the information. If a second person is not available to record data, videotaping while recording responses is a way of checking the therapist's data.

Functional Ability

An integral part of the sensorimotor treatment process is the patient's functional ability. Stimulation is provided the patient, followed by helping the patient use the body parts for whatever functional activity the patient is capable of doing. Prior to beginning the treatment program, evaluate the functional ability of the patient. Obtain as much information as possible from parents, teachers, and others who care for the patient, and by personal observation of the patient. Answers to the following questions about the patients' abilities and interests will be helpful in developing a treatment plan.

Does the patient react to auditory stimulation? What reaction does the patient make? Is the reaction different to different kinds of auditory stimulation, indicating an awareness of differences, or is the reaction the same? Is there hypersensitivity to auditory stimulation?

Does the patient react to visual stimuli? What types of visual stimuli elicit a response? What kind of response is made?

What gross-motor abilities does the patient have? Is the patient ambulatory? If not, is the patient able to move in some fashion? Is mobility purposeful? What fine-motor abilities does the patient have? What active, spontaneous upper extremity movements are possible? Are movements purposeful? Does the patient bring either hand to the mouth? Does the patient reach out and touch objects or surfaces? Does the patient rub surfaces? Does the patient hold objects? Does the patient reach out for people?

Does the patient relate to any person or persons? What behaviors are shown when the particular person or persons are visible or audible to the patient? Does the patient turn toward the person? Does the patient smile or vocalize in response to the favorite person?

What are some foods, objects, or other stimuli that the patient prefers? How is that preference expressed? What stimuli are distasteful or disliked by the patient. How is that dislike expressed?

When the patient is alone, what behavior is shown? What behavior is shown by the patient when disengaged, but in a group in the living area? Are any repetitive, stereotypical behaviors shown? What are these behaviors? When do these behaviors occur? Does the patient have any play behaviors? When and under what circumstances do these play behaviors occur? What are the behaviors? Does the patient have expressive language? Are there any meaningful gestures? What receptive language is present?

Does the patient have any independent bathing, feeding or dressing skills? Does the patient assist with any part of these activities done for him or her? Are there particular times or circumstances during which the patient shows more interest or skill in these activities?

What cognitive abilities does the patient show? What changes in cognitive ability have teachers and others noted?

Answers to these and related questions will help plan treatment objectives, methods, and target dates for achieving objectives.

Treatment Planning

The initial important goal of the treatment is the reduction or extinction of the SIB. The subsequent, and perhaps the most important, goal is to enable the patient to interact in his or her environment in such a way that the patient feels in control of some part of his or her own destiny.

Sensorimotor treatment for SIB is based on providing specific sensory and motor stimulation to the body systems, primarily the tactile, vestibular, and proprioceptive systems. The therapist plans the kind and amount of stimulation based on the location of self-injury, how the injury is accomplished, and on the evaluation of the patient's level of functioning and patient needs.

Determine which area of self-injury is most important to treat. Usually the most important area of injury is the one that creates the greatest threat to the patient. Injury to the eye, which can result in a detached retina, may be the most important for one patient. Head banging, which can result in an intracranial hemorrhage may be the most important area of self-injury for another patient.

The therapist should keep in mind body areas that require protection from injury during treatment. These areas also need to be stimulated carefully and consistently.

Sensorimotor Treatment Techniques

In planning treatment procedures, the therapist should be familiar with a variety of ways to provide sensorimotor stimulation. The following suggests ways to provide gross- and fine-motor stimulation, tactile stimulation, vestibular stimulation, and proprioceptive stimulation. The various kinds of stimulation and the specific techniques used in treatment are discussed separately, but in actual treatment they are seldom used in isolation.

Gross- and Fine-Motor Stimulation

Gross- and fine-motor stimulation refers to the physical movement of the body and body parts so that the body as a whole and the joints are moved and assume different positions. If a patient is unable to actively move his or her own body, the therapist will need to provide and guide the movements. The patient's postural reactions, such as righting and equilibrium reactions, neurodevelopmental level and physical and medical condition need to be considered in planning gross- and fine-motor stimulation. The purpose of motor stimulation is to facilitate or elicit purposeful movements. The aim is to teach the patient patterns of movement used in self-care, in play activities, and other purposeful and functional skills. Initial passive movement of the body may need to be given to provide tactile, vestibular or proprioceptive stimulation which the body would normally receive if the patient spontaneously made such movements.

For example, the therapist might give motor stimulation by rolling the patient from back to right side and back, and then to the left side and back, if the patient is immobile except for some side to side head movements and some distal upper extremity movements. Other parts of the body might be passively moved by the therapist in the beginning of the treatment process to introduce the patient to movement.

If the patient has enough upper extremity movement and hits his or her head, movement of the head, tactile stimulation, and vestibular stimulation might be the appropriate stimulation early in the treatment process. Stimulation can be provided by placing the patient prone over a large therapy ball and rolling the patient forward so the head is lower than the body and rolling back so the feet touch the floor; repeat this movement a determined number of times. Massage of the hand and scalp and hair brushing provide tactile stimulation to the head being injured and to the hand used to hit the head.

Observe the patient's oral motor abilities. Does the patient voluntarily open the mouth in anticipation of food presentation? Does the patient protrude the tongue to lick a piece of ice presented in front of his or her mouth? Does the patient have tongue control for movements to either side, up and down, and to protrude and retract the tongue? Does the patient swallow? Does the patient have jaw control and jaw movements needed for eating?

The combination of upper extremity motor ability and oral motor ability can be used to teach the patient self-feeding. Since one of the basic needs of every person is nourishment, teaching self-feeding skills is one of the top priorities in any treatment program. Elements of self-feeding movements can be used as motor stimulation in the treatment of SIB. The immediate gratification from the food—the sensory stimulation to the olfactory, visual, gustatory, tactile, and motor systems—makes the eating process a natural way to provide stimulation. In many cases, SIB will decrease during mealtime.

Gross- and fine-motor stimulation will depend upon the particular patient's developmental state, functioning ability and needs.

The Treatment Process

The patient is treated as a whole, even though only one area of the body might be the area of self-injury.

The tactile, vestibular, proprioceptive, and kinesthetic (movement) stimulation impact on the total person. These somatosensory stimulations affect body systems which work in concert with each other. It is difficult to isolate a single form of stimulation and provide a patient with only one type of stimulation. However, one kind of stimulation may be emphasized at one time during the treatment process and one part of the body may receive emphasis at another time during certain phases of the treatment process. It is important to remember the interrelationship of the somatosensory systems and the interrelationship of the various stimuli to each other and to the body. For example, if a patient is rolled on a floor mat by the therapist for vestibular stimulation, the hands of the therapist on the patient's body provide tactile stimulation at the same time. If joint movement occurs, stimulating surrounding tendons and ligaments, and if muscles receive deep stimulation during the rolling, the body is provided proprioceptive stimulation. The movement of the body provides kinesthetic stimulation during the rolling process.

As treatment progresses, the therapist is guided by observations of the patient's responses to the input of stimuli from the therapist. A thorough understanding of normal neurophysiological development and psychosocial development as well as keen observation skills will aid the therapist in adjusting the treatment techniques to the patient's various and often unpredictable responses.

When some upper extremity movement can be made, the self-inflicted injury is usually done with one or both hands. Motor stimulation of the upper extremities should be given as early as possible in the treatment program. Manual guidance can be given to help the patient hold toys and begin hand washing. Teaching the patient to hold objects and learn purposeful play movements, such as holding rhythm sticks and rubbing them together, is often useful. This process can be expanded to holding a fingernail brush and brushing the hand or any part of the upper extremity and may progress to using the brush during hand washing. The patient may be able to progress to holding a hairbrush and brushing the head, to combing the hair and to brushing the teeth.

The ability to hold objects in the hand to play or perform some self-care activity provides tactile stimulation to the body. Using the hands for purposeful activities is incompatible with using the hands for self-injury.

Basic Guidelines

- Do not let the patient injure you. Obtain permission to use measures to protect yourself before working with an aggressive patient.
- Do not let the patient injure himself or herself during the treatment program.

- Use a firm "No!" and try to prevent any SIB if it can be done safely.
- Work only to the patient and therapist's tolerance.
- Plan to treat the patient at the same time during the day, in the same location.
- Plan a routine and maintain the basic routine until change is noted.
- Introduction of new procedures may increase SIB.
- If SIB decreases or continues to increase after three consistent sessions, alter the procedure.
- Handle the patient with firm, definite touch.
- Speak to the patient in a definite, but gentle manner. Make short meaningful comments. Avoid extraneous comments.
- Speak to the patient before touching. This is especially important for a blind patient.
- Tell the patient about his or her positive qualities when appropriate.
- Use nursery rhymes and hand play when appropriate.
- Sing or hum quiet rhythmical tunes when appropriate. This is often helpful during gentle rocking, rolling, or swinging.
- When possible, place the patient on a mat or onto textured covered equipment which will increase the tactile input to more parts of the body.
- Talk to the patient about the beginning and the end of each activity and about the end of the treatment session to help the patient anticipate the change to occur. For example, "I will rub this part one more time," or "Let's put on your shoes so you can go." Even if the patient is said not to be able to understand, or is said to be blind or deaf, the therapist's reactions and comments give the patient a clue to the change about to occur. In many cases, it is unknown how much the patient understands, sees, or hears.
- Record events after each treatment session. If videotaping services are available, videotape the initial and last session, and as many other treatment sessions as feasible.

Initial Session

Take the patient to the designated location. If it is possible to place the patient on the mat, do so. Begin in a sitting position unless the patient is unable to sit. A sitting position for both therapist and patient allows more stability and control of the patient while the therapist provides tactile stimulation to the upper part of the patient's body.

Apply tactile stimulation to the body part used for injury. Usually the dominant hand is used for most of the injury. Stimulate the entire extremity as described in Chapter 3. Stimulate the other extremity in the same way.

If the patient uses another part of the body for injury, stimulate that body part. For example, the patient may hit with the dominant hand and also bite the nondominant hand or arm. After the extremity is stimulated, stimulate the area around the mouth. When possible stimulate inside the mouth by using ice which can be licked or by brushing the teeth and gums.

Next, stimulate the body parts that are injured. If these areas are swollen, bruised, bleeding, or appear tender to the touch, use tactile stimulation that will soothe the area. For example, if the area around the eye is bruised and swollen, a cool, damp cloth gently applied, removed, and reapplied might be the most appropriate tactile stimulation. An area that has been scratched open may also be stimulated in a similar way. Ice, if carefully applied for one to two seconds, two to three times, is often an effective tactile stimulation. The area surrounding the bruised or scratched area can then be stimulated with gentle and firm pressure by the fingertip.

Make it clear to the patient that SIB is unacceptable during treatment. A firm "No!" and physically blocking the attempt at SIB should be used at each SIB attempt. For many patients this procedure used a few times is sufficient for the patient to avoid SIB during treatment. Some patients will raise the hand to hit, but will stop in the middle of the act if the therapist's hand is placed between the patient's raised hand and the area the patient expected to hit.

If the patient is aggressive as well as self-injurious, use extreme caution to avoid being injured. Patients who are self-injurious and aggressive often have unclean, unmanicured fingernails which add to potential danger to the therapist. It makes sense to use hand washing, nail clipping, and other self-care activities as soon as possible to provide stimulation.

The length of time for the first few sessions will vary. The treatment should be terminated at the therapist's discretion. Five minutes of somatosensory stimulation may be the appropriate therapy for the first few sessions. Increase the amount of time for subsequent sessions up to a maximum of 30 minutes.

Subsequent Treatment Sessions

Maintain a routine. It is important for the patient to have some expectation of what will happen. Be consistent in the intensity of basic tactile stimulation. Gradually increase areas of stimulation. Gradually add other types of stimulation.

Be consistent in showing disapproval of the patient's attempts at self-injury. Be consistent in showing disapproval of the patient's attempts at aggressive acts toward the therapist.

When adaptive responses are seen, incorporate those responses in self-care or play activities. For example, hand movements can be manually guided to purposeful hand play while the therapist recites or sings nursery rhymes such as "Patty Cake" or "Pease, Porridge Hot." Or, manually guide the patient's hand to hold a fingernail brush and brush the hand or fingernails.

Later the patient can be taught to use the fingernail brush during hand washing at the sink.

Continue to incorporate purposeful self-care and play activities into the treatment. Use activities and objects that provide tactile and proprioceptive stimulation which the patient can apply to his or her own body whenever possible.

Patient Progress

Changes in the patient should be seen within five sessions. SIB may fluctuate. Increased SIB often occurs after a longer period between treatment sessions, such as after a weekend if the treatment sessions are routinely Monday, Wednesday, and Friday.

Observe carefully and record after each treatment. Changes may be subtle or questionable. Record what is observed and what is felt to have been observed. All information will be helpful in later analysis of the treatment. Recording the therapist's feelings is often helpful to motivate the therapist to continue a very difficult and stressful treatment process.

Subtle changes may show that the treatment has a positive effect on the patient, even though the SIB continues. The patient may make eye contact or increase the gaze into the therapist's eyes. Sighing by the patient indicates relaxation and comfort. The tone of vocalization may change. The distressed whiny sound emitted prior to treatment may change to a more relaxed cooing sound. The intensity of SIB usually decreases. During subsequent treatment sessions less time is usually required to stop the SIB displayed at the beginning of the treatment session. The patient may extend the hand or leg to have the body part stimulated. These small changes indicate potential for further changes and are important to observe and document.

Discontinuation of Treatment

The decision to discontinue treatment depends on the particular situation. It is not always related to the extinction of the SIB. In some residential facilities, when the SIB has been reduced or extinguished by the therapist, other staff are responsible for further programs for self-care, play, or education. In a school setting the discontinuation of treatment may occur because of the end of the school term. Another reason for discontinuation can be the need for the therapist to treat other patients. Staff shortage and the therapist's feelings and interests in the program are realistic reasons for discontinuation of treatment programs, since the demand on the therapist can be stressful and physically difficult.

After discontinuation of treatment, an ideal situation would enable the primary therapist to be available to other staff and family for any needed assistance. Rarely is this ideal situation seen.

Case Reports

Highlights of three patients treated by the author or her staff are given. All three were nonverbal, severely or profoundly mentally retarded, institutionalized individuals with varying degrees of mobility. It is hoped that this sampling will assist the reader in individualizing the treatment procedure to the particular patient.

Darlene

Darlene, age 10, weighed 43 pounds and was legally blind with cataracts bilaterally. She was nonambulatory. She was diagnosed with cerebral spastic paraplegia. She was routinely restrained in a wheelchair during her waking hours. She wore a restraint jacket made of heavy canvas, with three ties in the back. Each sleeve had four two-inch-wide pockets from the wrist to above the elbow into which four wooden slats were inserted to prevent elbow flexion. Cotton mittens were tied at her wrist to further assure that she would not scratch body parts. Her eyes were the primary area for self-injury. One Monday, when Darlene was brought to the treatment area, her eyes were swollen shut, the surrounding area was severely bruised and lacerated. During the weekend, when fewer ward staff were on duty, another child apparently removed the slats in Darlene's jacket. Before staff members realized the situation, Darlene had already caused serious injury to herself.

Darlene had a self-stimulating behavior of retaining saliva in her mouth and voluntarily slowly letting the saliva dribble. Her bib and dress were usually soaked from the time she was bathed and dressed after breakfast to midmorning.

Darlene screamed, cried, and physically resisted being moved, touched, or handled in any way. Although diagnosed spastic paraplegia, she had voluntary flexion and extension of her lower extremities. She was able to kick her legs as a means of protecting herself from being touched. She also resorted to biting a person who tried to touch or move her.

Since there was so much resistance to being touched, combined with crying, screaming, hyperventilation, and aggression in spite of her frail physical condition, treatment was initiated cautiously. She was left in her wheelchair in her restraints and treated in the therapist's office. Initially pressure touch was applied around her mouth, pressure touch in a circular motion at her temples, and slow downward stroking on her throat, ending with pressure upward on her throat at the base of her tongue to facilitate swallowing. Swallowing became automatic after 3 weeks. Retention of saliva was extinguished, and the resistive behaviors also stopped.

The resistive behaviors were displayed at the beginning of each new procedure. As Darlene accepted stimulation on her face, the upper extremities were stimulated. The procedure was similar to that described in Chapter 3. As Darlene gradually accepted the stimulation, she started extending her arm to the therapist upon arrival at the treatment room, to have her mittens removed and her hands stimulated. Hand play was done following stimulation. The hand play consisted of manually guiding Darlene in the motions of "Patty Cake". Occasionally the therapist delayed the hand play to observe Darlene's reaction. She would reach out for the therapist's wrists and begin the movement with the therapist's hands. She soon began making rhythmical "uh'uh" vocal sounds to accompany the therapist's voice reciting the rhymes and songs.

Stimulation to the lower extremities again elicited the screams, crying, and aggressive behavior. As the stimulation was imposed upon her, she gradually accepted the stimulation and apparently found it pleasurable. She learned to predict that the lower extremities were stimulated following hand play, and would put out her foot and place it on the therapist's lap to have her shoes and socks removed.

Treatment was discontinued when the goal of extinction of SIB was reached and generalized to the ward area. Prior to treatment, three or four staff members were needed to restrain Darlene in order to bathe her. Following treatment she could be bathed without other staff holding her extremities to prevent self-injury. Gradual weight gain began after automatic swallowing was accomplished. The ward staff were able to teach Darlene to feed herself and to place her in regular clothing without restraints over a period of one month following extinction of SIB. Her parents, who faithfully visited each Sunday, were elated to see the changes occurring.

Mary

Mary was a 12-year-old nonambulatory girl who could scoot around on her buttocks. She was diagnosed as having hypothyroidism. Her parents reported that she used to say some words, was more alert, and had crawled about their home. In the institution, she sat wherever she was placed. She scratched, pinched herself, and pulled her hair repeatedly. She had two (½" to ¾" diameter) open, bleeding wounds on her scalp. She had numerous open, bleeding scratches on her scalp, face, arms, and legs. She had many scratches in varying stages of healing.

Treatment consisted of pressure touch on the scalp around the open wounds and a massaging motion with the finger pads on the entire scalp. The spine was stroked from the base of the skull downward as described earlier in this chapter. Her face, arms, and legs were given firm stroking and pressure stimulation. Open, bleeding areas were stimulated with ice and cold turkish towel applications. Her fingernails were clipped. Her hands were washed at each treatment. When her scalp started healing, her scalp was brushed with a hairbrush. A toothbrush dipped in weak saline solution was used to brush her gums, inside of her cheeks, and her tongue.

Mary's tongue constantly hung from her mouth. Facilitation techniques for tongue retraction were used, but were ineffective. After discussion with Mary's parents, the therapist raised questions about Mary's medication. It was found that Mary's medication for hypothyroidism needed adjustment.

Treatment for SIB was discontinued after three months when she stopped scratching, pinching her skin, and pulling her hair. Ward staff were requested to continue combing and brushing her hair regularly, brushing her teeth, engaging her in hand play, and making toys available to her. After her medication was changed and stabilized, she became more alert and mobile. She scooted about to get toys, became interested in other children on the ward, and would even get a toy and place it on another child's lapboard.

Brian

Brian was a thin, passive, nonambulatory 9-year-old boy. His chest was 26" and his waist measured 36" to 43". He swallowed air and retained it (aerophagia). He routinely held the dorsum of his hands near his mouth and moved his head in a swaying side to side movement to lightly rub his lips against his hands.

Treatment was done on a floor mat and began with touch pressure around his mouth and on his hands. He was placed lying on his side with the therapist at his back and rocked slowly from side to back. Rocking was done first with one side on the mat, then the other side on the mat. He was so passive that he needed to be placed in each new position. An aim of the treatment was to put him into positions which would elicit postural reactions from him. He was placed supine, the therapist kneeling near his buttocks. The therapist grasped each of his thighs just above his flexed knees and flexed his hips as far as possible. This movement was repeated slowly three to five times. He was rocked in prone on a large therapy ball or over a carpeted barrel to facilitate protective responses. He was placed in sitting and given an unexpected sideward push at the shoulder to elicit protective responses. He continued to hold his hands near his mouth rather than respond automatically to changes threatening his body position when he was in a sitting position. Emphasis was placed on getting him into the quadruped position. Gradually he was able to stabilize himself in the quadruped position and eventually to move forward in this position. This was done by placing Brian's legs on either side of the kneeling therapist's trunk, the therapist supporting his thighs and hips with her hands and arms and gently pushing him forward. Brian had to move his hand forward or lose his balance. He was also placed straddled on the seat of a horse-shaped tubular frame with casters. His hands were manually held around the tube and he was helped to move about. He eventually learned to use his feet to move himself on the "ride-'em-horse."

Brian responded to the vibration or sound of the piano. At each session the therapist spent a few minutes at the piano since Brian seemed to get pleasure from placing his hands on the piano as it was played. His facial expression changed during this time from that of little expression to one of occasional smiles. Gradually, rather than taking him to the piano, the therapist left him on the mat and went to the piano, while encouraging him to come to her. He would eventually crawl to the piano and sit near her feet with his back to the piano, or would kneel with his hands on the edge of the keyboard.

Brian's therapy was discontinued when aerophagia was controlled and his waist measurement was consistently around 28". Ward staff were requested to continue engaging Brian in physical movements and play, and to begin teaching him some self-help skills.

The preceding and other self-injurious and self-stimulating behaviors were extinguished in other individuals by means of similar somatosensory stimulation. The patients continued without SIB or self-stimulating behaviors as they learned to participate in play and self-care activities. These cases were treated prior to the author's published case study of Edna (Lemke, 1974) and the study described in Chapter III. Others are encouraged to try intervention techniques with persons with SIB using the methods described.

Chapter V

DISCUSSION

James Prescott (Boynton, 1974), a developmental neuropsychologist at the National Institute of Child Health and Human Development, National Institutes of Health, stated that the effects of somatosensory deprivation in childhood could be seen in the violent and aggressive behaviors in puberty. He believed there was less body touching and body movement of infants in Western cultures compared to other cultures where babies are carried around on the mother's body even as the mother attended to other work.

If inadequate somatosensory stimulation is seen in infants and children who are not taken from their families and placed in institutions, it seems reasonable to suspect that there is inadequate somatosensory stimulation for institutionalized, mentally retarded children who have physical disabilities limiting their mobility. Since these children cannot be aggressive to others as a way of getting needed stimulation, it may be reasonable to suspect that the self-injury is a means of providing their own stimulation.

Prescott (Boynton, 1974) stated that extreme somatosensory deprivation caused alterations in the physical characteristics of the brain so that there were fewer dendritic branches. Fewer dendritic branches result in fewer contacts between brain cells. Mechanical functioning of the brain's cells and its electrical activity can also be altered by somatosensory deprivation. The neurotransmitter substance responsible for communication between brain cells can also become abnormal due to the sensory deprivation. Adequate amounts of somatosensory stimulation can reverse some of the abnormal changes, providing there were no permanent structural changes.

A case study of a 19-year-old severely self-injurious girl was reported by Lemke (1974) in which the self-injury was successfully extinguished over a six-month period by using somatosensory stimulation. The length of time was due to many days when therapy was not possible due to the patient's hospitalization for an infected finger and the therapist's other obligations. The actual time spent in therapy was 38½ hours over the six-month period. The patient remains institutionalized, but the staff and the patient's mother report that she remains free of self-injury.

Success with the above patient and other unreported cases leads the author to believe that certain individuals, accidentally or cognitively, learn how to provide some self-stimulation in an otherwise meaningless, deprived environment. The individuals seem to learn that they can use the self-stimulating or self-injurious behavior to manipulate and even control environmental effects on their person. Some possibly learn that self-injury results in some response. The response can be attention from another person, loosening of the restraints, a diaper change, movement, auditory stimulation, or a change in body position.

Although it is felt that all types of somatosensory stimulation are needed to reduce SIB and maintain reduction, the treatment reported in the case study (Lemke, 1974) is not always possible. Since tactile stimulation is basic to all other forms of somatosensory stimulation, the effect of tactile stimulation on SIB was studied (Hirama, 1981). If it could be shown that even a small amount of added tactile stimulation during the daily handling of self-injurious individuals made a difference in the behavior, perhaps attitudes and management of these individuals would also change.

The description of two years of managing one 8-year-old self-injurious girl by May, Gilbert and Ostler (1981) is reminiscent of similar situations in most institutions for the mentally retarded. The short, unsuccessful trials at various treatment procedures, the inconsistencies in handling, and the staff resentments are too frequently repeated. A practical way of meeting the needs of the self-injurious individuals as well as those of direct care staff is needed.

That the individuals need stimulation, that SIB may initially serve to meet that need, and finally that the behavior may be maintained by caretakers' attention to the behavior was proposed by Edelson (1984). Jan et al., (1983) suggest that the eye-pressing in visually impaired children may have a physiological explanation in that the self-stimulation occurs when the demand of the brain for meaningful visual information is not adequately met.

Owahki, Brahlek, and Stayton (1973) studied the preference for vibration or visual stimulation in 30 mentally retarded children. They found greater preference for vibratory stimulation. They felt that children with lower mental ages preferred passive touch, which is oriented toward bodily sensations, and that their study provided evidence of the reinforcing qualities of vibratory stimuli. The researchers noted that passive touch or tactile stimulation preceded active touch, which is oriented toward the object's quality.

When given toys, self-injurious individuals were found to automatically use the toys to self-stimulate the injured areas (Favell, McGimsey, and Schell, 1982). This study provides some credence to this author's treatment procedures of providing stimulation to the area being injured as well as providing general body stimulation and then teaching the individual self-care skills which provide alternate sensory activities. The physiological, psychosocial, and neurodevelopmental needs of the individual with SIB need further study.

We frequently hear that we cannot take the giant leap from animal study and apply that knowledge to human treatment, but the findings of Harlow and Harlow (1962) and Montegu (1962) should be taken seriously in planning treatment of SIB. Interestingly, Fox (1981), a practicing veterinarian, uses findings from deprivation studies on human infants to strengthen his argument that massage and "tender loving touch" is essential for the well-being and normal growth and development of socially dependent animals. Fox states that he was skeptical about the benefits of massage until he had various types of massage, including Shiatsu (Namikoshi, 1969; Namikoshi, 1974), done to his body; he later trained to be a massage therapist.

In summary, there is much that is unknown about SIB. We cannot take a narrow view as we try to develop better treatment and management procedures. I have presented my experiences and knowledge as clearly as I am able. I realize there are gaps in my presentation. Perhaps others who work with individuals with SIB can help confirm, reject, or fill in the gaps in this presentation.

Appendix

TREATMENT TO REDUCE
SELF-INJURIOUS BEHAVIOR

GENERAL PROCEDURE

1. Begin each session with a verbal greeting, "Hello _____" while smiling and attempting eye contact if eye contact is lacking.
2. Remove any physical restraint for the part to be stimulated.
3. Do not talk during the tactile stimulation phase.
4. Stimulation will be applied with tips of index and middle fingers of hand(s). The stimulation will be gentle but firm enough to temporarily indent the skin.
5. Stimulate the two sides of the body at the same time when simultaneous stimulation is indicated.
6. Count time in seconds ("1001" equals one second).
7. End each second with "Goodbye _____" while smiling and attempting eye contact.

SPECIFIC STIMULATION PHASE I

Face:
1. Simultaneously stroke from outer edge of each eye to hairline 3 times.
   (Total time: 3 seconds)

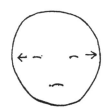

2. Simultaneously stroke from outer edge of lips up to temples 3 times.
   (Total: 3 seconds)

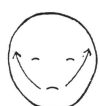

3. Simultaneously stroke from outer edge of lips to ears 3 times.
   (Total: 3 seconds)

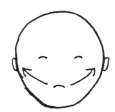

4. Simultaneously stroke from ear to outer corner of lips 3 times.
   (Total: 3 seconds)

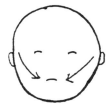

5. Place palm of one hand on top of head. Use index and middle fingertips of other hand, press above and below lips, one second each spot as numbered.
(Total: 8 seconds)

6. Simultaneously stroke from ear to collarbone 3 times.
(Total: 3 seconds)

7. Simultaneously stroke from edge of chin to collarbone (on both sides of esophagus).
(Total: 3 seconds)

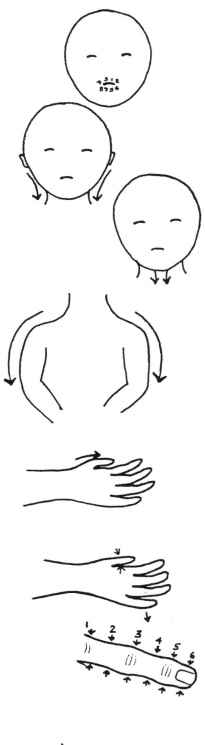

Shoulder:
1. Simultaneously stroke shoulder to elbow with palms 5 times. Duration of each stroke should be 3 seconds.
(Total: 15 seconds)

Upper Extremities:
1. Hold wrist with one hand. Individually stroke each digit from base to top. Hold digit laterally with thumb and first finger. Duration of each stroke should be 3 seconds. Repeat other hand.
(Total: 30 seconds)

2. Alternate a squeezing and releasing motion on each digit, moving from base to tip. Hold digit laterally with thumb and first finger, one second for each spot as numbered. Repeat other hand.
(Total: 60 seconds)

3. Cup palm in one hand. Stroke the forearm surface from wrist to elbow using fingertips 3 seconds per surface as numbered. Repeat other arm.
(Total: 30 seconds)

4. Cup palm in one hand. Alternate a squeezing and relaxing motion on each arm from wrist to elbow. Hold the arm in a palmar grasp. Duration for each squeeze-release motion should be 2 seconds. Repeat other arm.
(Total: 20 seconds)

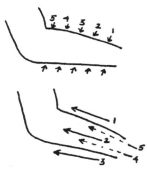

Functional Activity:
Follow tactile stimulation to face, shoulders, and upper extremities with some type of functional hand activity. The specific activity will depend upon the functional level and interest shown by the subject. Examples of activities are:

1. Manually guide subject's hands in clapping.

2. Manually guide subject's hands in applying lotion to hands, forearm, and/or face.

3. Encourage subject to handle objects such as textured cloth and toys.

4. Encourage subject to play with toys and/or games.

SPECIFIC STIMULATION PHASE II

Lower Extremities:
1. Stabilize the foot with one hand. Alternate a squeezing and releasing motion on each leg, working upward from ankle to knee. (Caution: Do not go above knee.) Duration for each squeeze-release motion should be 2 seconds at each spot.
(Total: 40 seconds)

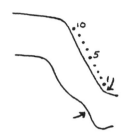

2. Stabilize the foot with one hand. Stroke the sole of each foot from the base of the toes to the heel 3 times. Duration for each stroke should be 3 seconds.
(Total: 18 seconds)

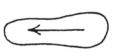

3. Stabilize the foot with one hand. Individually stroke the lateral surface of each toe from base to tip. Duration for each stroke should be 2 seconds.
(Total: 20 seconds)

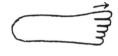

4. Stabilize the foot with one hand. Alternate a squeezing and releasing motion on each toe from base to tip. Hold toe laterally with thumb and first finger 3 seconds for each toe.
(Total: 30 seconds)

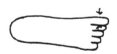

Functional Activity:
End tactile stimulation of lower extremities by providing some proprioceptive input. Example: If there are no contraindications, have subject bear weight, applying pressure downward from knees or hip with feet on a solid surface, or facilitate pushing the feet against a solid surface such as the therapist's hands or body.

1. If there are no contraindications, have subject bear weight on lower extremities.

2. If the subject cannot bear weight, position the foot against a stable surface with knee joint flexed. Apply pressure downward from knees (or stabilize knee joint and apply pressure upward from the soles of the foot).

SIB Response Form

NAME _____ # _____ DATE _____

Evaluator

_____

Instructions: On the line, write a descriptor, such as poke, bite, hit, scratch, for the SIB response.

HEAD	_____ R _____ L	
FOREHEAD	_____ R _____ L	
TEMPLE	_____ R _____ L	
EAR	_____ R _____ L	
NECK	_____ R _____ L	
TRUNK	_____ R _____ L	
SHOULDER	_____ R	
UPPER ARM	_____ R	
FOREARM	_____ R	
WRIST	_____ R	
HAND	_____ R	
THUMB	_____ R	

FINGERS:

1 _____ R
2 _____ R
3 _____ R
4 _____ R
5 _____ R

EYE _____ R _____ L
CHEEK _____ R _____ L
NOSE _____ R _____ L
MOUTH _____ R _____ L
LIP _____

JAW _____ R _____ L
CHIN _____ R _____ L

SHOULDER _____ L

UPPER ARM _____ L

FOREARM _____ L

WRIST _____ L
HAND _____ L
THUMB _____ L

FINGERS:

1 _____ L
2 _____ L
3 _____ L
4 _____ L
5 _____ L

CHEST _____

ABDOMEN _____

GENITALIA _____

THIGH _____ R _____ L

LEG _____ R _____ L

FOOT _____ R _____ L

TOES _____ R _____ L

SIB Response Form

NAME _____ # _____ DATE _____

Evaluator

Instructions: On the line, write a descriptor, such as poke, bite, hit, scratch, for the SIB response.

HEAD _____ R _____ L

FOREHEAD _____ R _____ L

TEMPLE _____ R _____ L

EAR _____ R _____ L

NECK _____ R _____ L

TRUNK _____ R _____ L

SHOULDER _____ R

UPPER ARM _____ R

FOREARM _____ R

WRIST _____ R

HAND _____ R

THUMB _____ R

FINGERS:

    1 _____ R

    2 _____ R

    3 _____ R

    4 _____ R

    5 _____ R

EYE _____ R _____ L

CHEEK _____ R _____ L

NOSE _____ R _____ L

MOUTH _____ R _____ L

LIP _____

JAW _____ R _____ L

CHIN _____ R _____ L

SHOULDER _____ L

UPPER ARM _____ L

FOREARM _____ L

WRIST _____ L

HAND _____ L

THUMB _____ L

FINGERS:

    1 _____ L

    2 _____ L

    3 _____ L

    4 _____ L

    5 _____ L

CHEST _____

ABDOMEN _____

GENITALIA _____

THIGH _____ R _____ L

LEG _____ R _____ L

FOOT _____ R _____ L

TOES _____ R _____ L

References

Allen, K.E., and Harris, F. R. (1966). Elimination of a child's excessive scratching by training the mother in reinforcement procedures. *Behavior Research and Therapy, 4,* 79–81.

Aronfreed, J., and Reber, A. (1965). Internalized behavioral suppressive and the timing of social punishment. *Journal of Personality and Social Psychology, 1,* 3–16.

Azrin, N. H., Gottlieb, L., Hughart, L., Wesolowski, M. D., and Rahn, T. (1975). Eliminating self-injurious behavior by educative procedures. *Behavior Research and Therapy, 13,* 101–111.

Azrin, N. H., Kaplan, S. J., and Foxx, R. M. (1973). Autism reversal: Eliminating stereotyped self-stimulation of retarded individuals. *American Journal of Mental Deficiency, 78,* 241–248.

Bachman, J. A. (1972). Self-injurious behaviors: A behavioral analysis. *Journal of Abnormal Psychology, 80,* 211–224.

Bailey, J., and Meyerson, L. (1970). Effect of vibratory stimulation on a retardate's self-injurious behavior. *Psychological Aspects of Disability, 17,* 133–137.

Baumeister, A. A., and Baumeister, A. A. (1978). Suppression of repetitive self-injurious behavior by contingent inhalation of aromatic ammonia. *Journal of Autism and Childhood Schizophrenia, 8,* 71–77.

Baumeister, A. A., and Forehand, R. (1973). Stereotyped acts. In: N. R. Ellis (Ed.) *International Review of Research in Mental Retardation.* New York: Academic Press.

Beckwith, B. E., Coulk, D. I., and Schumacher, K. (1986). Failure of Naloxone to reduce self-injurious behavior in two developmentally disabled females. *Applied Research in Mental Retardation, 7,* 183–188.

Berkson, G., and Mason, W. A. (1963). Stereotyped movements of mental defectives: III. Situation effects. *American Journal of Mental Deficiency, 68,* 409–412.

Birnbrauer, J. W. (1968). Generalization of punishment effects: A case study. *Journal of Applied Behavior Analysis, 1,* 201–211.

Brawley, E. R., Harris, F. R., Allen, K. E., Fleming, R. S., and Peterson, R. F. (1969). Behavior modification of an autistic child. *Behavior Science, 14,* 87–97.

Bright, T., Bittick, K., and Fleeman, B. (1981). Reduction of self-injurious behavior using sensory integrative techniques. *The American Journal of Occupational Therapy, 35,* 167–172.

Buchar, B., and King, L. (1971). Generalization of punishment effects in the deviant behavior of a psychotic child. *Behavior Therapy, 2,* 68–77.

Buchar, B., and Lovaas, O. I. (1968). Use of aversive stimulation in behavior modification. In: M. Jones (Ed.) *Miami Symposium on the Prediction of Behavior, 1967: Aversive stimulation.* Coral Gables, FL: University of Miami Press.

Cain, A. C. (1961). The presuperego turning inward of aggression. *Psychoanalytic Quarterly, 30,* 171–208.

Carr, E. G. (1977). The motivation of self-injurious behavior: A review of some hypotheses. *Psychological Bulletin, 84,* 800–816.

Carr, E. G., Newsom, C. D., and Binkoff, J. A. (1976). Stimulus control of self-destructive behavior in a psychotic child. *Journal of Abnormal Child Psychology, 4,* 139–163.

Cautela, J. R., and Baton, M. G. (1973) Multifaceted behavior therapy of self-injurious behavior. *Journal of Behavior Therapy and Experimental Psychology, 4,* 125–131.

Cleland, C. C., and Clark, C. M. (1966). Sensory deprivation and aberrant behavior among idiots. *American Journal of Mental Deficiency, 71,* 213–254.

Corbett, J. (1975). Aversion for the treatment of self-injurious behavior. *Journal of Mental Deficiency Research, 19,* 79–95.

Corte, H. E., Wolf, M. M., and Locke, B. J. (1971). A comparison of procedures for eliminating self-injurious behavior of retarded adolescents. *Journal of Applied Behavior Analysis, 4,* 201–213.

Crabtree, L. H., Jr. (1967). A psycho-therapeutic encounter with a self-mutilating patient. *Psychiatry, 30,* 91–100.

Davidson, P. W., Kleene, B. M., Carroll, M., and Rockowitz, R. J. (1983). Effects of Naloxone on self-injurious behavior: A case study. *Applied Research in Mental Retardation, 4,* 1–4.

DeCatanzara, D. A., and Baldwin, G. (1978). Effective treatment of self-injurious behavior through a forced arm exercise. *American Journal of Mental Deficiency, 82,* 433–439.

DeLissovoy, V. (1963). Headbanging in early childhood: A suggested cause. *Journal of Genetic Psychology, 102,* 109–114.

Dorsey, M. F., Iwata, B. A., Ong, P., and McSween, T. E. (1980). Treatment of self-injurious behavior using a water mist: Initial response suppression and generalization. *Journal of Applied Behavior Analysis, 13,* 343–353.

Dorsey, M. F., Iwata, B. A., Reid, D. H., and Davis, P. A. (1982). Protective equipment: Continuous and contingent application in the treatment of self-injurious behavior. *Journal of Applied Behavior Analysis, 15,* 217–230.

Duker, P. (1975). Behavior control of self-biting in a Lesch-Nyhan patient. *Journal of Mental Deficiency Research, 19,* 11–19.

Edelson, S. M. (1984). Implications of sensory stimulation in self-destructive behavior. *American Journal of Mental Deficiency, 89,* 140–145.

Favell, J. E., McGimsey, J. F., and Schell, R. M. (1982). Treatment of self-injury by providing alternate sensory activities. *Analysis and Intervention in Developmental Disabilities, 2,* 83–104.

Fisher, S. (1974). *Body Consciousness.* New York: Jason Aronson, Inc. pp. 20–40.

Fox, M. W. (1981). *Dr. Michael Fox's Massage Program for Cats and Dogs: A new approach to pet health care and fitness.* New York: New Market Press.

Frankel, F., Moss, D., Schofield, S., and Simmons, J. Q. (1976). Case Study: Use of differential reinforcement to suppress self-injurious and aggressive behavior. *Psychological Reports, 39,* 843–849.

Green, A. H. (1967). Self-mutilation in schizophrenic children. *Archives of General Psychiatry, 77,* 234–244.

Harlow, H. F., and Harlow, M. K. (1962). Social deprivation in monkeys. *Scientific American, 207,* 136–146.

Hirama, H. (1981). *The effect of tactile stimulation on self-injurious behavior.* Unpublished dissertation. Dissertation Abstracts International, 42(3-A), 1097 ISSN: 04194209. Ann Arbor, MI: University Microfilms International.

Hoefnagel, D. (1965). The syndrome of athetoid cerebral palsy, mental deficiency, self-mutilation and hyperuricemia. *Journal of American Deficiency Research, 9,* 69–74.

Holburn, C. S., and Dougher, M. J. (1985). Behavioral attempts to eliminate air-swallowing in two profoundly retarded clients. *American Journal of Mental Deficiency, 89,* 524–536.

Holburn, C. S., and Dougher, M. J. (1986). Effects of response satiation procedures in the treatment of aerophagia. *American Journal of Mental Deficiency, 91,* 72–77.

Jacobs, H. E., Lynch, M., Cornick, J., and Slifer, K. (1986). Behavior management of aggressive sequela after Reye's syndrome. *Archives of Physical Medicine Rehabilitation, 67,* 558–563.

Jan, J. E., Freeman, R. D., McCormick, A. Q., Scott, E. P., Robertson, W. D., and Newman, D. E. (1983). Eye-pressing by visually impaired children. *Developmental Medicine and Child Neurology, 25,* 755–762.

Kelly, J. A., and Drabman, R. S. (1977). Generalizing response suppression of self-injurious behavior through an over-correction punishment procedure: A case study. *Behavior Therapy, 8,* 468–472.

Lane, R. G., and Dormath, R. S. (1970). Behavior Therapy: A case history. *Hospital and Community Psychiatry, 21,* 150–153.

Lemke, H. (1974). Self-abusive behavior in the mentally retarded. *The American Journal of Occupational Therapy, 28,* 94–98.

Lesch, M., and Nyhan, W. L. (1964). A familial disorder of uric acid metabolism and central nervous system function. *American Journal of Medicine, 36,* 561–570.

Lester, D. (1972). Self-mutilating behavior. *Psychological Bulletin, 78,* 119–128.

Lourie, R. M. (1949). The role of rhythmic patterns in childhood. *American Journal of Psychiatry, 105,* 653–660.

Lovaas, O. I., Freitag, G., Gold, V. J., and Kassorla, I. C. (1965). Experimental studies in childhood schizophrenia: I. Analysis of self-destructive behavior. *Journal of Experimental Child Psychology, 2,* 67–84.

Lovaas, O. I., and Simmons, J. Q. (1969). Manipulation of self-destruction in three retarded children. *Journal of Applied Behavior Analysis, 2,* 143–157.

Luiselli, J. K. (1986). Modification of self-injurious behavior: An analysis of the use of contingently applied protective equipment. *Behavior Modification, 2,* 191–204.

Matione, F. F. (1977). Reducing self-abuse in a severely retarded adolescent male through the use of positive reinforcement and fading. *Special Children, 4,* 32–38.

May, A. E., Gilbert, T., and Ostler, E. (1981). Self-injurious behavior: A case study. *British Journal of Mental Subnormality, 27,* 74–81.

Measel, C. J., and Alfieri, P. A. (1976). Treatment of self-injurious behavior by a combination of reinforcement for incompatible behavior and over-correction. *American Journal of Mental Deficiency, 81,* 147–153.

Merbaum, M. (1973). The modification of self-destructive behavior by a mother-therapist using aversive stimulation. *Behavior Therapy, 4,* 442–447.

Mikkelsen, E. J. (1986). Low-dose Haloperidol for stereotypic self-injurious behavior in the mentally retarded (correspondence). *The New England Journal of Medicine, 315,* 398–399.

Mizuno, T., and Yugari, Y. (1974). Self-mutilation in the Lesch-Nyhan syndrome. *Lancet, i,* 761.

Montegu, A. (1971). *Touching: The human significance of the skin.* New York: Harper & Row, pp. 214–252.

Mutter, A., Peck, D., Whitlow, D., and Fraser, W. (1975). Reversal of a severe case of self-mutilation. *Journal of Mental Deficiency Research, 19,* 3–9.

Myers, J. J., and Deibert, A. N. (1971). Reduction of self-abusive behavior in a blind child by using a feeding response. *Journal of Behavior Therapy and Experimental Psychiatry, 2,* 141–144.

Namikoshi, T. (1969). *Shiatsu: Japanese finger pressure therapy.* Tokyo: Japan Publications, Inc.

Namikoshi, T. (1974). *Shiatsu Therapy: Theory and practice.* Tokyo: Japan Publications, Inc.

Nyhan, W. L. (1976). Behavior in the Lesch-Nyhan syndrome. *Journal of Autism and Childhood Schizophrenia, 6,* 235–252.

Ohwaki, S., Brahlek, J. A., and Stayton, S. E. (1973). Preference for vibratory and visual stimulation in mentally retarded children. *American Journal of Mental Deficiency, 77,* 733–736.

Peterson, R. F., and Peterson, L. R. (1968). The use of positive reinforcement in the control of self-destructive behavior in a retarded boy. *Journal of Experimental Child Psychology, 6,* 351–360.

Picker, M., Poling, A., and Parker, A. (1979). A review of children's self-injurious behavior. *The Psychological Record, 29,* 435–452.

Primrose, D. A. (1979). Treatment of self-injurious behavior with a GABA (gamma-aminobutyric acid) analogue. *Journal of Mental Deficiency Research, 23,* 163–173.

Ragain, R. D., and Anson, J. E. (1976). The control of self-mutilating behavior with positive reinforcement. *Mental Retardation, 14,* 22–25.

Repp, A. C., and Deitz, S. M. (1974). Reducing aggressive and self-injurious behavior in institutionalized children through reinforcement of other behaviors. *Journal of Applied Behavior Analysis, 7,* 313–325.

Romanczyk, R. G., and Goren, E. R. (1975). Severe self-injurious behavior: The problem of clinical control. *Journal of Consulting and Clinical Psychology, 43*, 730–739.

Rutter, M. B. (1966). Behavioral and cognitive characteristics of a series of psychotic children. In: J. K. Wing (Ed.) *Early Childhood Autism*. London: Pergamon Press.

Sandman, C. A., Datta, P. C., Barron, J., Hoehler, F. K., Williams, C., and Swanson, J. M. (1983). Naloxone attenuates self-abusive behavior in developmentally disabled clients. *Applied Research in Mental Retardation, 4*, 5–11.

Saposnek, O. T., and Watson, L. S. (1974). The elimination of the self-destructive behavior of a psychotic child: A case study. *Behavior Therapy, 5*, 79–89.

Schroeder, S. R., Peterson, C. R., Solomon, L. J., and Artley, J. J. (1977). EMG feedback and the contingent restraint of self-injurious behavior among the severely retarded: Two case illustrations. *Behavior Therapy, 8*, 738–741.

Seegmiller, J. E., Rosenbloom, F. M., and Kelley, W. N. (1967). Enzyme defect associated with a sex-linked human neurological disorder and excessive purine synthesis. *Science, 155*, 1682–1684.

Shear, C. S., Nyhan, W. L., Kirman, B. H., and Stern, J. (1971). Self-mutilative behavior as a feature of the deLange syndrome. *Journal of Pediatrics, 78*, 506–509.

Silberstein, R. M., Blackman, S., and Mandell, W. (1966). Autoerotic headbanging. *Journal of the American Academy of Child Psychiatry, 5*, 235–242.

Singh, N. H., and Pulman, R. M. (1979). Self-injury in the deLange syndrome. *Journal of Mental Deficiency Research, 23*, 79–84.

Smolev, S. R. (1971). Use of operant techniques for the modification of self-injurious behavior. *American Journal of Mental Deficiency, 76*, 295–305.

Stainback, W., Stainback, S., and Dedrick, C. (1979). Controlling severe maladaptive behavior. *Behavior Disorders, 4*, 99–115.

Tanner, B. A., and Zeiler, M. (1975). Punishment of self-injurious behavior using aromatic ammonia as the aversive stimulus. *Journal of Applied Behavior Analysis, 8*, 53–57.

Tate, B. G. (1972). Case study: Control of chronic self-injurious behavior by conditioning procedures. *Behavior Therapy, 3*, 72–83.

Tate, B. G., and Baroff, G. S. (1966). Aversive control of self-injurious behavior in a psychotic boy. *Behavior Research and Therapy, 4*, 281–287.

Tierney, D. W. (1986). The reinforcement of calm sitting behavior: A method used to reduce the self-injurious behavior of a profoundly retarded boy. *Journal of Behavior Therapy and Experimental Psychiatry, 17*, 47–50.

Weiher, R. G., and Harman, R. E. (1975). The use of omission training to reduce self-injurious behavior in a retarded child. *Behavior Therapy, 6*, 261–268.

Wells, M. E., and Smith, D. W. (1983). Reduction of self-injurious behavior of mentally retarded persons using sensory-integrative techniques. *American Journal of Mental Deficiency, 87*, 664–666.

Williams, C. E. (1974). Self-injury in children. *Developmental Medicine and Child Neurology, 16*, 88–90.

Young, J. A., and Wincze, J. P. (1974). The effects of the reinforcement of compatible and incompatible alternative behaviors on the self-injurious and related behaviors of a profoundly retarded female adult. *Behavior Therapy, 5*, 614–623.